INSPIRATION FOR THE WEARY THERAPIST

Inspiration for the Weary Therapist is a companion for the modern practitioner. Addressing a diverse audience and written by a master clinician and supervisor, *Inspiration for the Weary Therapist* helps modern therapists traverse the complicated landscape of practicing therapy in the age of COVID-19.

Instead of a heavy, theoretical approach that can leave the already exhausted therapist feeling more overwhelmed, *Inspiration for the Weary Therapist* guides readers through challenging professional situations, soothes them during upsetting clinical moments, and encourages them to keep going during changing times. Rather than teaching mental health professionals how to practice, this book helps them believe in themselves again and reconnect with their confidence as clinicians through increased self-compassion and personal growth.

This practical and helpful guide is essential reading for all mental health practitioners who are searching for inspiration and motivation and who want to reconnect to what it means to be a therapist.

David Klow, LMFT, is the author of *You Are Not Crazy: Letters From Your Therapist* and the founder of Skylight Counseling Center in Chicago.

"David Klow has offered us a supportive and generous book from the trenches. Although he too is wrestling with the role of the therapist during this time of massive global upheaval, he has found a way to convey to us a deep well of both empathy and leadership. This is no small feat! He writes simply (because he knows we are weary), but he writes thoughtfully (because he knows we cannot indulge simplistic formulations at a time like this). This is a book every clinician needs to have on their shelf."

Alexandra H. Solomon, PhD, *adjunct faculty at the School of Education and Social Policy at Northwestern University, licensed clinical psychologist at The Family Institute at Northwestern University, and host of the "Reimagining Love" podcast.*

"*Inspiration for the Weary Therapist* is a delight to read! It richly delivers on Klow's promise to fill the gaps in a therapist's formal training, combat burnout, and offer practical suggestions from his many years of clinical work and supervision. Transcending models of therapy, the book covers the important topics of boundary setting, self-care, offering advice, and many more that bedevil practitioners. Therapists of all experience levels will find pearls of wisdom and telling clinical examples in these pages."

Arthur Nielsen, MD, *clinical associate professor of psychiatry and behavioral sciences at the Feinberg School of Medicine at Northwestern University, and the author of* A Roadmap for Couple Therapy *and* Integrative Couple Therapy in Action.

"*Inspiration for the Weary Therapist* is just that and more. David Klow, a superb therapist and supervisor, offers precisely the sort of book that early career therapists and students in the mental health fields need. Sagaciously, Klow's overarching theme lies in helping readers to find and retain their own therapeutic voice, even in these trying times. Yet, this book also brilliantly offers an almost endless repository of therapeutic tools as well as practical guidance about the pragmatics of working as a therapist. Filled with clinical wisdom and well-chosen vignettes, this is clearly a book every therapist can learn from and should be required reading for every beginning therapist."

Jay Lebow, PhD, ABPP, LMFT, *clinical professor, senior scholar, and senior therapist at The Family Institute at Northwestern University.*

INSPIRATION FOR THE WEARY THERAPIST

A Practical Clinical Companion

David Klow, LMFT

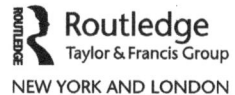

Routledge
Taylor & Francis Group

NEW YORK AND LONDON

Cover image: © Getty Image

First published 2023
by Routledge
605 Third Avenue, New York, NY 10158

and by Routledge
4 Park Square, Milton Park, Abingdon, Oxon, OX14 4RN

Routledge is an imprint of the Taylor & Francis Group, an informa business

Library of Congress Cataloging-in-Publication Data
Names: Klow, David, author.
Title: Inspiration for the weary therapist : a practical clinical companion
  / David Klow, LMFT.
Description: Abingdon, Oxon ; New York, NY : Routledge, 2022. | Includes
  bibliographical references and index.
Identifiers: LCCN 2022002469 (print) | LCCN 2022002470 (ebook) |
ISBN 9781032251844 (hardback) | ISBN 9781032251820 (paperback) |
ISBN 9781003283164 (ebook)
Subjects: LCSH: Psychotherapists--Job stress. | Counseling
  psychologists--Job stress. | Mental health counselors--Job stress.
Classification: LCC RC451.4.P79 K56 2022 (print) |
LCC RC451.4.P79 (ebook) | DDC 616.89/14--dc23/eng/20220211
LC record available at https://lccn.loc.gov/2022002469
LC ebook record available at https://lccn.loc.gov/2022002470

ISBN: 978-1-032-25184-4 (hbk)
ISBN: 978-1-032-25182-0 (pbk)
ISBN: 978-1-003-28316-4 (ebk)

DOI: 10.4324/9781003283164

Typeset in Joanna
by KnowledgeWorks Global Ltd.

For Manny & Goldie

CONTENTS

ACKNOWLEDGMENTS

This book came about organically, through a series of talks with fellow therapists at my practice, Skylight Counseling Center, in Chicago. Without the hardworking and dedicated staff, past and present, at Skylight, this book would not exist. It is their deep desire to help others and be good at their craft that pulled forth the material for this book. I want to thank the team at Skylight who have shown such devotion to their clients during stressful times. I am blessed to be surrounded by such inspiring individuals who show me how to put their care for others into action.

I especially want to acknowledge Natalie Jeung and Claire Argall, who helped me create this book. Natalie used the video recordings of the talks with the staff and carefully edited them down to the core themes that were most salient. Natalie's attention to detail and clinical knowledge were such assets in creating this project. Natalie handed the edited videos off to Claire, who carefully transcribed each one and gave me the core written material to work on, which would eventually become this book. I couldn't have done this project without Natalie and Claire. Thanks so much to you both!

I also want to thank Alexandra Solomon, Art Nielsen, and Jay Lebow, who provided support, encouragement, and feedback about the manuscript. Your wisdom, experience, and care have been crucial to my development as a clinician and author. Being in consultation with you and the other remarkable couples counselors in our group has helped me clarify how I think about the work we do.

I stand on the shoulders of great therapists and supervisors and can only hope to pass along some of the knowledge and wisdom that I have learned from them. Chief among these mentors are Linda Rubinowitz and Marina Eovaldi, who helped shape me as a clinician and showed me what a truly loving supervisor can be like. Thank you for believing in me and getting me started in this field. Thanks also to the many supervisees that I have worked with over the years who helped me learn how to be a better therapist. From training you, I learned how to clarify the work that I do.

Thank you to Anna Moore at Rutledge for your willingness to believe in this project and, from Day 1 understanding what I was trying to accomplish with this book. Your ideas and suggestions helped fine-tune the material so that it could reach more therapists out there who need the support and encouragement. I appreciate your ongoing support in getting this book to publication.

Thank you to my wife, Angelica, who has shown me how to open my heart to real love and connection with another human being. I am not only better at being a therapist with you in my life, I am a better person because I am with you.

Last but not least, I want to acknowledge all of the therapists working today who are burnt out, overwhelmed, and struggling with their own lives but still find a way to be fully present and care deeply for their clients. When I sit down for a session, especially if I'm not feeling up to it that day, I think about you also sitting down with your clients at the same time. You may have a lot going on in your lives, but you know how to clear that to the side and care for the other human being in front of you. It's not easy work, and I hope that this book can give back just a little something so that you can keep going. I am glad that you are out there!

INTRODUCTION

Times are tough for therapists. We find ourselves in the midst of many perfect storms. Global changes, social unrest, tremendous upheaval, and trauma in the lives of our clients and our own besiege our clinical path. We put our hearts on the line in session and bleed openly with our clients. We throw ourselves into the mud with them and their messy lives. We work tirelessly to bring hope to those who are bereft and give direction to those who are lost.

It is a beautiful, noble, and worthwhile effort: our life's work. Yet often, it is a slog. Our clients report a bit of progress, but then things fall apart. Our efforts to get through to them come up short. We can become lost and hopeless ourselves, watching people we have grown to care about continue to suffer and struggle.

In these moments, we turn to our supervisors or case consultants. We ask them to help us better understand the client and their presenting problem. We look for new methods or ways of thinking about the case. Supervision becomes the one place where we can talk openly about the work and find insights into how we can be more effective.

Quite often, however, supervision can become stale. We keep talking about the same cases, and the supervisor keeps offering the same perspective. Worse yet, supervision can turn into a game of Whack-a-Mole

DOI: 10.4324/9781003283164-1

where we reactively try to solve the issue of the week. Instead of growing professionally and developing our clinical skills, supervision often turns into a place where we try to fix the most stuck cases and solve our clients' endless problems. This often leaves the therapist in a reactive, hopeless place facing an onslaught of daily clinical problems.

As clinicians, we need to go beyond case consultation. We need to get to find inspiration and reconnect to what it means to be a therapist. As mental health practitioners, we talk about cases in supervision, but we often do not address our personal, professional, philosophical, and even spiritual development. We stay stuck in the details of cases instead of looking more expansively at trends in how we practice. Instead of supervision on our cases, we need inspiration and companionship that we can take to heart and share with our clients.

The essence of an inspired caseload is lived experience. To become a good therapist, we need to learn from our clients. When something goes wrong with a case, we can look at what happened, but we also need to go beyond the specifics. We need to discover the broader themes that show up across our practice. If, for instance, upon losing a case, we realized that the client felt misunderstood, then we could look at what it really takes to understand a client and for them to feel understood. We do not want to stop with just the case at hand. We want to develop ourselves as clinicians.

Moving beyond case consultation and into professional development is a vital and often missing component of clinical supervision and often leaves the supervisee feeling weary and alone. Having been a clinical supervisor in agency, educational and private practice settings for over 15 years, I have found professional development to be an essential aspect of supervision. I am certainly interested in the details of my supervisee's cases. I want to help them handle specific clinical issues and enable them to figure out where to go with their cases. Addressing what to do in session is one very important part of supervision, yet there is so much more available.

There is another gear of supervision that has to do with developing ourselves as people. We must go further than the case consultation part of supervision and dive right into the big themes that show up in the therapy room. We need to resource the therapist at their roots, so they do not get bogged down in the details of their endless cases.

There are so many weary therapists out there burdened and overwhelmed by the gravity of the current human condition. My hope with this book is to cumulatively nourish our work so that we don't have to go it alone. Rather than solving all of the tough cases we face on a regular basis, I hope to provide a deeper sort of inspiration and companionship that reaches further into the heart of our work. By getting to the source of the issues that befall us, I trust that we might find new perspectives and solutions to our most vexing cases.

As a cisgendered, straight, white male, I hold excessive privilege along with the power that comes with being a therapist. I am working on how my biases and privileges as a white man might impact how I practice, what I write, and how I understand what those around me are experiencing. Yet even with working on it, I carry tremendous blind spots and often default to the white-centered biases of our field. I am working on unpacking this through what Dr. Jennifer Mullan calls decolonizing therapy.[1] Yet there is a lot of work to do, and there are certainly aspects of this book that may miss the mark. My hope, though, is that the messages in this book can serve all clinicians of all identities and inspire and uplift all of us that do this important work. My hope is that this book can be a practical clinical companion so that it supports the work of therapists everywhere.

There are, of course, many ways that clinicians practice. There is not one therapy. We each have our approaches and our preferred methods and theoretical backgrounds. This book does not claim to cover how every therapist practices. Rather it aims to address some of the common factors that cut across disciplines. The topics in the book typically exist in many of the modalities and approaches to doing therapy. A Cognitive Behavioral therapist might approach some of these topics in ways that an Emotionally Focused therapist would not. Regardless of the background or approach, some common factors exist in the practice of mental health counseling, and the topics addressed here hope to cross the boundaries of different kinds of therapy. While therapies do differ, the ideas and advice in the book can apply for the Cognitive Behavioral therapist as well as the Emotionally Focused therapist or Dialectical Behavioral Therapy practitioner, even if they apply the ideas through the lens of their own perspective. This book does not aim to address how to practice such models, but it does consider the differences experienced in coming from different perspectives.

Inspiration for the Weary Therapist started as a series of clinical conversations and talks with my staff at Skylight Counseling Center in Chicago. We started what we called "Supervision for the Soul" as a way to move beyond case consultation into the heart of what we do as clinicians. I ran these talks and recorded the contents of what I spoke about with my staff. Their questions clarified and elicited information about supervision that I would not have been able to articulate otherwise. We took the recordings, edited them down, and transcribed them. I built upon the transcription, polished and edited it, and turned it into this book in the hopes of sharing the material with clinicians everywhere, helping them cope with the struggles of practicing today.

The reason why I call this book *Inspiration for the Weary Therapist* is that it aims to reach into the deepest part of what it means to be a therapist and uplift those of us who are worn down by the work. Instead of having to go it alone, my hope is that this book is a companion of sorts that provides encouragement, ideas, new perspectives, innovative ways of working, and practical tips that set up the modern therapist to practice for a lifetime. If this book can inspire you, the therapist, then you might inspire your clients. If this book can provide some nourishment, then you will have just a little bit more to offer others. I hope that some of this book reaches the roots of you who are so you will continue to flourish.

Introduction Bibliography

1   https://www.drjennifermullan.com/

1

PRACTICING DURING UNCERTAIN TIMES

This chapter looks at how practicing therapy has changed in recent times. As the world changes around us, so does our work in session. Learning how to practice remotely during a pandemic, making sense of how social and political unrest change how we practice, and being prepared to guide people through uncertain times has become essential to being a clinician today. This chapter helps modern practitioners find some clarity about practicing during uncertain times.

Rethinking therapy

We need to rethink what therapy looks like. The image of a therapist sitting comfortably in their chair with the client across the room on the couch, clutching a box of tissues or a throw pillow, cups of tea sitting on side tables with a clock auspiciously placed within the therapist's trained and caring gaze, might be a thing of the past. We need to let go of some of our assumptions about what therapy is and what it will become.

DOI: 10.4324/9781003283164-2

Many therapists never imagined doing mostly remote therapy, barefoot, family in the other room, client logging in from their parked car, testing the audio and video before finding a good connection, the clock prominently displayed in the window of our computer screen. Yet that is what therapy became in an instant during the COVID-19 pandemic, which in the United States took hold in March of 2020. The goal of creating a safe, contained space in which it was safe to look within had to adjust to larger global health factors. Both the client and the therapist's central nervous systems were better served being in separate spaces, not in the same room. Being together in session would have created too much arousal. If one person sneezed or coughed, or if the client said they were traveling, it would likely have been too distracting to allow for the tranquility of a normal, private therapy session.

Moving online became more effective. Confidentiality had to be reconsidered. Clients logging in from their bedrooms and bathrooms became the norm. Sometimes they would log on with a glass of wine in their hands, other times there was someone in the next room from them. All of the predictability and control of in-person therapy went away and was replaced by a mode of treatment that was the solution for pandemic life. At first, most therapists were unsure how to practice this way. Yet over time, they found creative solutions, discovered ways to adjust, and learned how to practice anew. This sort of adjustment was uncomfortable for most but also showed the resiliency of therapists who were dedicated to serving their clients.

Practicing during uncertainty is not something that is new for clinicians. There have been times over the years where therapists have had to forget everything that they knew, discard their training, and just practice from instincts. On 9/11 in the United States, therapists had no answers for what was happening but had to show up for their clients and help them through the fear and confusion. During political upheaval and social unrest, clinicians have needed to bravely face their own uncertainty and reactivity and be honest with their clients within the scope of therapy. While we might wish to focus our sessions on our clients' personal growth and development, there are times when we are called instead to help steady the ship on the changing tides of history.

Creating new boundaries

Learning how to practice during uncertain times is essential to being a therapist today. We have to be prepared for working in unexpected and unfamiliar situations. We also need to become comfortable controlling what we can and letting go of those things that are out of our control. Drawing a boundary around what is considered therapeutic is important but might also be changing. What we used to think of as out of bounds might now be acceptable if we wish to conduct therapy. We need to continually revisit what constitutes a *break* in the therapeutic boundary. Of course, confidentiality is essential. We need to maintain confidentiality if therapy is going to work. We also need to get clear about what we can guarantee is confidential and what is out of our control. While we choose a telehealth system that is compliant with the Health Insurance Portability and Accountability Act (HIPAA), we cannot guarantee that the client's end of the platform will be secure, especially if other people are nearby when they are speaking. I would never do an in-person therapy session at a coffee shop, yet I have had to do a few telehealth sessions in which the client was calling in from an outdoor patio at a cafe. It was clear that there were others around, but this was the most secure place they could find.

Our own work-life boundaries need to be reimagined as well. Where once we had clear boundaries about being at work versus being at home, in uncertain times, we find ourselves reexamining what our office looks like. During the COVID-19 pandemic, most therapists had to adjust to practicing from home, much like other people who had the privilege of working from home. Learning how to create the mindset for working with clients while one's family is in the next room was an adjustment for many clinicians. Redefining what the space is for therapy is a big part of practicing during uncertain times.

What helped for me was thinking about Rupert Sheldrake's notion of the extended mind.[1] In this notion, we understand the mind to extend beyond the body and make connections across space. Even if I were not in the same room as the client, perhaps our minds would form a sort of connection in the moment across the video screen or phone line. While I was much more accustomed to feeling a connection in person during sessions, it took some adjusting to recognize the meeting of the minds in a remote session. Over time, my intuitive clinical instincts got used to not being in the same room as the client and found their way into sessions in ways that felt quite comfortable and familiar.

Experiencing uncertainty alongside the client

What is typically not comfortable and familiar for most therapists is experiencing the same struggles as the client at the same time. Usually, we can hold space for our clients while they experience difficulties in their lives. Often we are not in the same exact experience with them. For instance, if they are going through a divorce or the loss of a loved one, unless we are also having our own divorce or loss at the same time, we can find perspective and perhaps even share our lived wisdom from our previous breakups or losses in life. Even if we are going through a divorce at the same time as the client, it is a separate situation, with different circumstances, and we might be able to find perspective so that we can be in a solid place to support the client. Usually, we can hold space for clients by finding parallels between their experiences and our own. For a client currently experiencing divorce or the loss of a loved one, we can find perspective or even share our wisdom from our own lived experiences of breakups or losses. With a global pandemic, for instance, we are in the same situation with the client. We are swimming in the same waters and might not have any answers, wisdom, or perspective to offer the client.

Experiencing the uncertainty of changing times alongside the client calls for a different sort of practice of therapy. We cannot reassure the client that everything will be alright, for we do not know if that is the case. We cannot stay a neutral observer of their struggles either because we are in the same boat. It would seem dishonest and disconnected if we did not acknowledge that we are having troubles with life's changes too. In fact, it might form more of a bond with the client if we can give them a bit of a sense of how we are in it with them. We, of course, won't make the session about us and our own pains, but we can find ways of indicating that we are working on managing life's uncertainties as well. Maybe we have some coping strategies, but that might be all that we can offer, other than our time and our presence in session.

In a way, we are redefining what the therapy hour is when we meet with a client during uncertain times. Our time and our presence might indeed be all that we have to offer. Trying to offer more would be forcing it, and it would also be unfair to ourselves. Why would we try to overdo it? If we are impaired in some ways by living through challenging and uncertain times, we need to downshift our expectations of what we can do and what is possible in therapy. If you are normally a therapy sports car that can run in fifth gear, you might only be able to make it into third gear when the world around you is chaotic and out of balance. Therapeutic third gear might not feel as fulfilling as fifth gear, where tremendous, measurable progress and insights are gained, but it is more realistic, efficient, and honest. Your clients will be better served by you being okay with just being present with them in the uncertainty of life than by you trying to conduct therapy as usual.

Self of the uncertain therapist

Practicing during uncertain times means that we will likely feel uncertainty. The self of the therapist that usually feels connected, passionate, open, curious, and kind might feel uncertain. When we are learning to become a therapist, there is uncertainty about how to practice and what to say in session. This is quite normal, and clients usually are able to tolerate working with us while we learn our craft. While this sort of uncertainty does not necessarily feel good for the developing therapist, it is different from that of a therapist living during uncertain times. When most everything that we know in our personal and professional lives is thrown on its head, it creates an inner sense of being untethered. The ground metaphorically moves beneath our feet, and it can be difficult to pay attention to anything other than finding solid footing.

In these sorts of situations, the uncertain therapist needs radically heightened self-care. We need to be okay with our work being the best that it can be, even if "best" is mediocre. Practicing mental health care during troubling times is frontline work. The collective trauma of our clientele and of humanity gets into us and amplifies our own trauma responses of the moment. Instant compassion fatigue and burnout result. Hearing horrible stories and people's lives falling apart session after session is unendurable. The empathic, sensitive therapist will absorb the weight of distress from their clients and get pulled under.

I heard from numerous seasoned therapists during the COVID-19 pandemic that, for the first time in their long careers, they thought about quitting. We might be able to withstand the suffering of our clients on a regular basis, but when everyone is suffering, including us, it causes the best of us to consider a career change. In these moments, increased self-care and a more realistic sense of what is possible in therapy need to be employed.

Surviving uncertain times

Banding together as therapists is also needed. Uncertain times often cause clinicians to feel alone and practice alone. The certainty of practicing alongside each other every day at the office, seeing one another for connection and consultation, can be taken away from us when our entire way of practicing is thrown upside down. Having to endure session after remote session alone in our home offices is not what we were trained to do. It does not match the spirit of the work of being with our clients in ways that are deeply felt and connected.

During these sorts of uncertain moments, we can imagine all of our fellow therapists simultaneously sitting down for their sessions with their cups of tea, readying themselves to be present, and holding space for their clients. We can count ourselves among them, understanding that we are not alone. We are part of a team of healers guiding our fellow humans toward a more holistic way of living on this planet. We can give ourselves a break and not feel like we have to figure it out or fix it ourselves. Others can help us. We can form teams of therapists that support our clients. We can find new ways of practicing that are more efficient, effective, and made for these times.

Reinventing how we do therapy is imperative during uncertain times. Uncertainty usually leads to something new. If we cling to old ways while the world changes around us, we get stuck in the past. Letting go of who we were and embracing the new therapist we are becoming might be the best way to gracefully move forward. We can do this.

Chapter 1 Bibliography

1   Sheldrake, R. (2003). *The Sense of Being Stared at, and Other Aspects of the Extended Mind*. London: Hutchinson.

2

REAL SELF-CARE: HOW TO AVOID BURNOUT

This chapter looks at how to nourish ourselves as therapists both in and out of session, especially in challenging life situations. We go beyond typical self-care and look at what it takes to avoid burnout as a clinician practicing today.

Being present while being in pain

Self-care is vital for therapists. We learn from very early on in our training that we need to take care of ourselves in order to care for others. Yet a deeper and more symbolic question emerges when we ask ourselves how to be present with others when we are in tremendous pain ourselves. When the care of self goes beyond managing day-to-day stress, how does one stay grounded and connected with clients when physical, mental, relational, or psychological pain is overwhelming? What does self-care look like when you are at a level of weariness and burnout?

DOI: 10.4324/9781003283164-3

Theoretically, as a healer (a wounded healer, perhaps), you do not have to be 100 percent well in order to help people. You do not have to have your life perfectly together in order to be a therapist. In fact, some of the best work I have done has been when I have felt completely broken. During some of my most overwhelming personal challenges, I have found that being a therapist can even help ground me. Physically, I have worked when I have had a cold and have learned where my line is in terms of needing a sick day. When life's challenges are too much, we need to know when to take a break.

Sometimes when life is too challenging, you can default back to doing more listening with clients because you need to have more of your attention on yourself in those moments. If you are in chronic pain, you have to know where your limit is, even if it is a movable line from week to week. You need to know what the indicators are of when you are not well enough to do the basics of being present, attuned, and thinking clearly. How much can your mind and body handle while still being able to do the basics? That is the crucial inquiry around burnout.

Nowadays, there are new modalities of therapy. I certainly struggle with the "therapist in your pocket" notion when the client can just text their therapist. I struggle a bit with remote therapy, too. There is something about being in the room with somebody and having that live, intimate exchange. It is palpable. Whether you are in person or doing remote therapy, the client needs to have an interaction with you as a live being. To make that happen, you need to be alive, inhaling and exhaling, in the moment with them. We need to be vital enough to actively give and receive.

When we are in a lot of pain, our output to input ratio will change. If we are guilty of giving too much to our clients and not receiving enough from our lives, then we need to change the way we think about healing so that we do not give out more than we take in. We have to be okay with simply being present with our clients. We do not have to move mountains and do their work for them. Sometimes in therapy, you have to care for yourself too. We have to focus on taking in our own life more in order to feel whole. Have your coffee in session. Sip it. Take in the light that's coming in the room. Our clients need us to be present and alive.

Our clients need us to travel more, too! Travel for some people might cause more stress, but for others, it can be a good practice of self-care. Something happens when we are on vacation. A mindset takes over: everything seems new, days feel longer. We can only be away from the office for a week, yet it can feel like a month. This mindset is difficult to replicate when we are at home, but if we craft a mindset of taking in the world anew everyday it can positively impact our presence in session.

To be a good therapist your mind and body need to say, "I'm glad to be here!" To be present, we need to be feeling pleasure. When we are in pain, it is easy to check out mentally. When we encounter other people's pain, it can be doubly difficult to remain present. We can benefit from looking more closely about how we feel about our relationship with other people's pain as well as our own. Finding a way to take care of ourselves and soothe our own emotional and physical pain can help with being present with our clients day after day.

What you need to be present

What will you need to be present in session even in the face of other people's pain? Do you need different cushions on your chair? Will always having food or tea with you help? How about comfy clothes? A blanket thrown over your legs? A little footstool? A fan in the heat of summer? You may need a whole little apothecary on the table next to you. Let's let that be okay. If it gets to where there is a lot of stuff on your table, just tell your clients what is going on. I think it is acceptable for a therapist to have a cup of something nourishing next to them in session.

You do not need to hide your pain from your clients. You can let clients know what you are going through. Clients benefit from having a full human being with them who is giving, receiving, experiencing joys, struggling, and even suffering. Giving yourself permission to be a full person that is comfortable in the therapy room allows you to be present. You are getting paid for your presence, so you need to cultivate it. If you are in pain, your presence is even more of a commodity. It needs to be harvested.

We need not clear everything out of our mind, be totally empty, and have no distractions in order to be present. I have seen new therapists who won't even move their gaze away from the client at all. That is too rigid. Instead, it helps to stay relaxed and open. Of course, don't check your phone. That would not be appropriate. For the most part, stay in your seat, but feel free to get up at some point. You urgently need to go to the bathroom during a session? You have permission to say, "I'm sorry, I have been having some stomach pains. I need to go to the bathroom." We don't need to override ourselves so that we are suffering in order to be present in session.

Giving requires receiving

To give to our clients, we also need to be adept at receiving. Receiving a breath, receiving a hug, receiving your food, receiving sunlight, receiving sleep, and receiving company with people are all simple ways of taking in life so that we have more to give to clients. Excessive giving can be a defense against receiving, as it can feel very vulnerable to receive.

In graduate school, we did an exercise where we had to feed each other pudding. It was horribly uncomfortable because it was so intimate. One person would feed the other, and the other would just receive, and then we would switch. When I was on the receiving end of being fed, it was very vulnerable because the feeder was also so uncomfortable. She fed me at too quick a pace when I was not yet ready for more food. She was uncomfortable and was teasing me with the food too. It was way too intimate, and she was in total control. When I was feeding, I felt more in control, but it was still a strange exchange to be feeding her. The idea of the exercise was that, as a therapist, we are in the position of feeding our clients, and they are on the receiving end of that giving.

This graduate school exercise made it very clear that it felt so much better to feed than to be fed. We have to keep that in mind in session. Our clients are in the role of being fed, and it does not always feel so good for them. They are in a powerless place and we are in control. To be more effective at our feeding and to understand the control and power we have therapists, we need to work on our ability to receive and remove any barriers to taking in life.

For instance, how do you receive gifts from clients when they give you a present to express their gratitude? We are supposed to give to our clients, but the tables turn when they give to us. It is important for us to be open in those moments and receive the gratitude that is being offered to us. Instead of saying, "Oh, thank you very much" and then putting the gift away, we might instead make a show of it and ceremonially receive what they bring us. Being fed by them in some way might help us be even more effective at feeding them overall.

The practice of being human

What we are positing here is that the therapist is a better agent of healing and change if they are able to receive nourishment and also nourish themselves. To be effective with the management of our client's pain, we have to respond to our own suffering with warmth; otherwise, we cannot practice deep compassion for others. When you give others a break for being a certain way, but you won't let yourself up be that same way, it is not real compassion. It is unnecessarily beating yourself up, thinking that you need to be strong in order to help.

It is human to be weak. There is an essential part of the therapeutic relationship in which strength on the part of the therapist is valued. We are essentially saying to our clients, "I am stronger. I can hold this space for you. You are not going to overwhelm me." The client wants to feel the therapist's strength. However, what if the therapist is not feeling strong? What if they convey something that says, "I am overwhelmed. I do not think I can handle all of your stuff."? This might not help the client feel safe. It might also replicate early wounds for them. There is the potential that if we are human and fragile that the client might not feel in capable hands.

In these situations, there is also the potential for something reparative to happen. The client may get to witness us having a bad day or struggling in our own lives while being completely capable of helping them. It exhibits a broader spectrum of possibilities in a healthy, human relationship. If I were having a tough time in my life, it would feel very weird to not let the client know what is going on. It can improve the therapeutic relationship to disclose a bit of what is happening in my life because it sends the message that our relationship is strong enough that I can share with them. I have been surprised that when I start telling them my story that the client might have just a few questions but then will smoothly shift back to what is happening in their life.

When you are more vulnerable with clients, you are sharing with them what it is to be human—that sometimes you are not always doing well. You acknowledge that the human experience is varied, that you are not ideal, but instead very human.

May the *person* you are be the same as the *therapist* that you are. May who you are in the therapy room be the same as who you are *outside* the room. You will feel way more at ease this way. Let your clients see you. They want to be seen, and they want to be able to see you. Remember that your ability to see others only goes as far as your ability to be seen.

3

EMPOWERING THROUGH LOVE: HOW TO IMPART STRENGTH TO OUR CLIENTS

In this chapter, we explore empowerment. How do we empower our clients, and what does that really look like in practice? There are no easy answers, but in essence, if we love and accept someone exactly as they are, if gives them the space and permission to grow into who they might become. We need to find ways to love our clients through the tough times and give them a glimpse at what it looks like to have someone who cares in their corner.

Our role is to empower

What does it look like to empower our clients? How do we effectively get them to step into the fullness of who they are and access the range of their strength and ability? Let's break down the mechanics of what it actually means to empower somebody else. What does that look like theoretically and in practice?

DOI: 10.4324/9781003283164-4

First, be sure that you are working to empower your client and not trying to solve their problems for them. A lot of times, we get caught up in the content that clients bring to session, and we try to fix their issues for them. Instead, what we should be doing is empowering them to find their own solutions. Solving the problem for them may relieve some of their distress, but it does not actually empower them to solve future life problems. When you think of what it means to empower your clients, what do you think about? What does that look like for you?

If we are not truly practicing personal power, we might not be able to instill empowerment in others. In our own power as a clinician, we must recognize how impactful it is to be a witness to our clients. Recognizing their strength, their brilliance, their wisdom, or their effectiveness can have a very empowering effect on them. You can feel confident knowing that one thing you can do is witness, acknowledge, and validate the client when they are functioning well. The confidence you have in your ability to do this can be infectious.

The health premise

Where does real empowerment come from? Is it something that a therapist can bestow upon their client? Or is empowerment an aspect of being human that needs to be cultivated? Often the therapeutic process is mistakenly driven by the desire of the therapist to have something happen, to feel like they are making something happen. Rather than letting the process unfold, the therapist pushes to see the client make changes in their life. They want to see that their work is making an impact through tangible results, such as the client moving out of an unhealthy living situation, leaving their abusive partner, or finally getting a job. If the client is not making tangible results, or if you are not sure what the results are, it is difficult to let the process simply unfold so that something authentically empowering can occur.

Instead of pushing for results, we could instead focus on the health premise. The health premise is the assumption that our clients are inherently healthy, yet there are forces outside of them that take that health away. They are fully capable, yet there are certain specific and real constraints to them being fully healthy or fully functional. With this perspective, we are not operating from a place of finding what is wrong with the client and trying to fix it. Instead, we take the approach that they have native wisdom, a built-in ability to find answers and get the most out of their lives, and we work to bring that to the forefront.

There is a seed within each client that needs germination. Something may be getting in the way of that germination, and the therapist's job is to remove that obstacle. For example, a client might express various thoughts and feelings that say, "I feel unsafe. I feel anxious. I feel alone. I've always been alone in this world, and nobody knows what I'm going through. Nobody has really been there for me or seen anything like this before." When a client is activated like that, they usually cannot simultaneously access their power, wisdom, abilities, or answers.

In the presence of a truly compassionate therapist who has done some of their own work on themselves, the client encounters something new. They might recognize that here is someone who has seen some things, who cares about people, who is willing to go there and willing to be there with them. This sort of presence can cause them to breathe and relax and have some part of their brain come online that they could not access when they were stuck in feeling alone. In this sort of encounter, we are not empowering them through a "rah-rah" pep talk. Instead, we are providing empowerment through a safe, soothing attachment relationship in which they can feel fully met and held.

This sort of therapeutic relationship can change the way that a client experiences relationships in general. So many clients get constantly pulled into the feeling that the other person is the problem or that their partner is doing something hurtful to them. This can quickly lead to feeling disempowered in their relationships. If we can get our clients to feel, even just a little bit, that relational change can occur and that they might be able to create some of that change, then they will get a sense of having more options in their life.

We help facilitate this shift in perspective by being with the client and loving them in a way they have not been loved by another person before. We believe in them—not necessarily because we believe in their personality but because we believe in humanity, and we know what is possible within each person. As we get to know them, we see things in who they are that reinforce our enduring belief in their innate power.

Reframe problems

Another way to empower a client is by reframing their issues into something that can be more easily transformed. A reframe is a type of intervention where we change the way a situation or idea is viewed. A client might see a life experience in one way that might be limiting, and we work to change the context in which the experience is viewed so that it means something else. A reframe gives them a little bit of play and room to look at things differently. While that may be a basic therapeutic intervention, it can have a huge impact.

Creating new viewpoints and perspectives is a big part of therapy. Even the way we sit with clients can create new angles of looking at things. In the therapy room, I like it when my chair is off to the side a bit on an angle, and the client is looking straight forward. They are symbolically looking off into the distance at their life and their problem and I am looking at it from a different angle, off to the side, to help see it differently. As therapists, we look at our clients and their lives from a different angle and perspective, and that frees them up to look at it differently as well, especially when they are feeling hopeless. Feeling disempowered and feeling hopeless go hand in hand. A lot of people come to therapy saying, "This is happening to me, my life is happening to me. I'm suffering and struggling as a result of it, and I don't know what to do." Our job is to help them see their situation differently.

I have a client whose daughter went off to college for her first semester. His daughter has a history of anxiety, eating disorders, and body image issues. The father got a call from the daughter saying she was in the hospital for an episode of panic attacks and problematic eating. The father was not sure what to do, but he also felt guilty about not wanting to take action. He asked, "Is it horrible that I don't want to go out there? I actually like that my daughter is away at school in the hands of competent caregivers, rather than in my house."

He was worried that I would judge him for not wanting his daughter home. Yet my stance was that it is not horrible. It made sense that he wanted some space. He had been on a roller coaster with his daughter for years. He had been so "in" this with her daughter that it had been hard for him to even know how to navigate this situation. It had almost been easier with the daughter away at college, so he wasn't obliged to go charge over to the hospital.

My saying, "No, that's not horrible that you are feeling that way," changed his thinking about the situation. Now the father could reflect on his options on how to be most effective rather than sitting in guilt. Maybe he would be more powerful in how he intervened. He might be more powerful in the interaction if he were willing to embrace that it is okay to appreciate the distance, as otherwise, he might be operating out of obligation. This client was freed up to be more effective once he stepped out of judging his own interactions. It often takes the therapist's nonjudgmental stance to free the client up from their habitual, disempowering guilt.

Force versus power

We illuminate for a client that they have power in a situation by being powerful ourselves. Rather than being forceful in the room with them by trying to make something therapeutic happen, we transmit a sense of easy confidence when we trust in the power of the therapeutic process. In his 1974 Rumble in the Jungle match, Muhammad Ali famously used a technique called the rope-a-dope. In this approach, he would lean back on the ropes acting if he were cornered, and let his big opponent swing at him until he got exhausted. Once Ali's opponent, world heavyweight champion George Foreman, punched himself out, Ali was able to use his quickness to outlast the stronger opponent. In this case, Ali didn't meet force with force. He likely would have lost if he had. Instead, he found a cunning way to become more powerful in the ring.

When it feels as if we are in a hopeless, powerless situation, we can draw on Ali's example and find a creative way to assume some power. For instance, if someone in our life is intruding on a personal boundary, we would be meeting force with force by yelling at them and telling them off. Instead, it is more effective to invite them into a conversation, even get a little bit closer to them, so that we can get to the bottom of their intrusions and eventually back them off for good. If we can do this in our personal lives, then we should be able to set an example for our clients. The client can start emulating that in their own relationships.

How we align ourselves in the therapy room can convey a sense of empowerment. Showing our clients that we can honor the session by starting and stopping on time lets them know that there is power in boundaries. Showing them that we collect their agreed-upon fee for service demonstrates that we know the value of our work. Being available for them within the scheduled therapy session and not for ongoing phone or email conversations shows them that we won't give ourselves away. All of what happens in the therapy process is a chance to demonstrate how to be empowered. The goal is to have that be transmitted to the client and to imbue them with that empowerment.

4

HOW TO GO WITH THE FLOW

In this chapter, we look at the balance between spontaneity and order. As therapists, we need to have some semblance of control and order to our sessions so that they are contained. Yet a big part of the work we do is also being able to go with the flow and work with what shows up in the session. This chapter explores how to "go with it" and play with what shows up in the room, as well as how to manage various boundaries in session.

Going with the flow

As therapists, we provide structure, regularity, and reliability with clients. We hold boundaries. If we have a session scheduled at a certain time, we stick with the plan. If a client suddenly asks to bring their spouse into an individual session, and that spouse is in the waiting room with them, then we may not let that happen. A big component of what

DOI: 10.4324/9781003283164-5

we do is hold boundaries because it keeps our work with the client reliable. Yet there is an art to the practice of therapy that includes going with the flow.

A client of mine was recently talking about his relationship with his spouse and that he has been having a difficult time sharing more deeply with her because she is sometimes critical. She called him on the phone during the session, and he asked if I minded if he took the call. Normally, I would wonder why this person is taking a phone call in session and I might ask if they really need to take it. I would suggest that if it is not important that they should stay focused on the therapeutic work that we are doing.

In this case, for some reason, I said, "Sure, please feel free to take the call."

I was not sure why I did that, but I just went with it and let what was unfolding in the session occur. My client answered the phone and I could hear her voice on the other end. She asked him if he had picked up something for the kids and he said no. She replied that she was at the store and that she would happily take care of it. From where I was sitting, she sounded lovely and gracious on the phone and said some sweet things to my client.

I certainly had not planned for this to occur, but hearing my client's brief exchange on the call with his spouse gave me insight about their relationship. Had I not gone with the flow and encouraged him to answer the call, I never would have had this extra data. Once he hung up the phone, I asked him if the exchange on the call was unusual. He said no, and I commented that she sounded really nice in how she spoke with him. He remarked that she is a really sweet person and that is what she is usually like. It surprised me because he had been painting a picture of a very critical and unavailable person. The image that I had of her was based on what he had told me. Hearing her on the other end of the phone gave me another image. What he had been telling me was just a little piece of the story. Going with the flow of the session allowed me to get this extra data and opened up a whole new way that I might work with this client.

I had originally thought that for him to share more deeply with his spouse or be more affectionate with her would be a big stretch, since she sounded unavailable and unreceptive. Yet maybe in reality it was not as big of a stretch as it was in his perception. Maybe she was more open and receptive than he thought? Hearing his spontaneous call with her changed the way that we worked, and it happened because I just went with it.

Using spontaneity in sessions

Much like when my client answered his phone, something unexpected happens in session when you go with the flow. We also need to be prepared for the unexpected that happens on the boundary of therapy such as in the waiting room.

On another occasion, a different client wanted to bring their spouse into session without my knowing in advance. It did not make sense to me for the spouse to join the session, so I stuck to my boundary and encouraged us to wait. My gut feeling was that it would become more chaotic to have the spouse join the session without proper preparation on everyone's part. While I might have gotten more data if we did a couples session, I wanted it to be more structured and organized. Going with the flow did not make sense in this instance.

You may be surprised when you are expecting one person in your waiting room and find another. There is no manual for what you are supposed to do in these situations, and you have to rely on a split-second instinct of what you are supposed to do in the moment. One example is that an adolescent's parents may show up for the session because the child was sick, and they thought they could just meet with you individually. If you were not expecting to do a parent meeting that day, but all of a sudden, there they are in your waiting room, wanting to meet with you, then you have to think on your feet.

You may have to quickly check with yourself, and say, "I am sorry, I was not prepared for a session with you. I can't meet with you today."

This response might be appropriate, but it can also be quite rigid. The client might understand and respect your boundary, but they might also get upset by your turning them away and even charging them for a canceled session since the child did not attend. If you do let the parent into a session with you to talk about their child and you are not prepared, then it could cause even more problems. The session could go poorly and even more importantly, your adolescent client might not appreciate that you met with their parent without talking with them first. It could cause all sorts of problems if you go with the flow and let the parent in, yet it might also allow for some new insights about the family system. These are difficult calls to make. We can be guided ethically by our professional standards of care and also by our training. We need to make sure that we have proper training and credentialing to work with more than one person in the room should we include other members of the system. Attuning to levels of confidentiality and what we are required to do to manage boundaries can guide us case by case. We have to take that knowledge and think on our feet in the moment.

In many ways, the practice of therapy is inherently spontaneous. Cultivating spontaneity in our practice can really serve the work we do. We need to learn to trust spontaneity as a therapeutic tool. When do we use it and when do we stick with our plan? In session, in the moment, we choose what to say and what to do. There is a lot of improv in the work. We have to trust our instinctual reactions as they arise in response to the client's presentation. It often does not work to script a session or dictate exactly what the conversation will be. It is not natural that way. Newer therapists may like to prepare what they will talk about in the session with their clients. Yet that does not leave room for what the client wants to bring in. We can go with it for a while and then we steer the conversation back to topics that are more therapeutic.

It is not all or nothing. We do not have to be completely spontaneous and without structure, and we don't have to be fully rigid either. It is a bit like jazz, where there is a basic structure to the piece but then plenty of room for improvisation. We go with what a client is talking about, but that does not mean we have to stay with that topic the whole time. If my client who took the call during session had kept going, there would likely be a point where I would have had to ask him to get off the phone. I would want there to be a limit to this sort of spontaneous occurrence. Similarly, I would not have gone with it as far as having him put her on speaker so that I could talk with her too. Going with the flow does not mean that I am going to keep going with whatever is happening without setting a limit. I might go with it for a little while and then change gears back to where I think the therapeutic material is.

We just need to know our limits and also what our goal is with spontaneity. Could we see that at the end of the road of spontaneity is beauty? In our very programmed, organized, orderly lives, there is beauty in spontaneity. When we are spontaneous, we can actually find things that are more beautiful than we would have found otherwise.

Boundary of spontaneity and rigidity

On the other end of spontaneity is rigidity. For most of us, the problem is likely not that we are too spontaneous. It might actually be that there is too much rigidity in our practices. For instance, if you let that parent of the adolescent into session when they showed up without prior notification, how would you feel during that meeting? Would you feel like you are locked into a full session with them because you let them into your office? By letting them in, do you now have to do a full 50 minutes? Or could you talk with them for a 10-minute check-in and then politely ask them to leave? Being able to adjust on the fly and not feel trapped when a client compromises your boundaries can allow for more fluidity.

Rigidity and spontaneity may seem like a binary, but they are more of a spectrum. A healthy system has some permeability. It is not overly rigid or too diffuse. New therapists often need to rely on a rigid structure for therapy to work and for them to feel comfortable and held together. They may cling to rules learned in graduate school and their sessions can be too automated. This is understandable, as the practice of therapy is so multidimensional and unpredictable. Lack of structure would feel too chaotic. An overly structured therapy practice can prevent us from being adequately flexible and effective.

We can think of our families of origin as a way of understanding our relationship to boundaries and systems. Was your family of origin one with a rigid boundary around the system? What were the boundaries like within and around your family? Was it diffuse, people coming in and out with no predictability? Or was it very rigid? If we were raised in a system with semipermeable boundaries, where there was flow in and out the family but there was enough containment, then that might set us up nicely to handle boundaries in a healthy way as a therapist. Yet most of us likely came from a family system that was either too rigid or too diffuse in the boundaries. If this is the case for you, then it would make sense that there would be a learning curve around how to naturally handle therapeutic boundaries.

Creating boundaries in sessions

I have seen clients stop working with their therapist because they felt like they could dictate the terms of therapy too much. If we give the client carte blanche and free range to set the therapy how they want to, it doesn't necessarily mean that they will want to stay. Actually, some clients might stay because the therapist is quite clear and firm on the boundaries and the client feels well respected and taken care of because the therapist is able to say no.

Let us manage what we can. If we pay attention to how we start and stop sessions, we create the needed structure that holds up in-session spontaneity. Starting your in-person sessions, you might think about the door to your office. If you know that your next client is a boundary pusher and likes to pop their head in before the session starts, then close your door before the session. You could keep your door closed until you are absolutely ready to start. When you open the door, if you have just one person coming into session, you might hang back by the doorway and invite them in.

If you have a family coming in to see you, then you need to be careful about how you manage the door. If you are anticipating the entire family coming in from the waiting room, then you might simply open the door for them to all come in. But if you are anticipating just some family members entering while others wait in the waiting room (for instance, a parent waits in the waiting room while you see their adolescent child), then you can slip out of your office, close the door behind you, walk into the waiting room, and greet the family so that they all don't come charging in when you open the door. The door is your way of controlling who is in the in-person session and who is not. A closed door sends a message that the person is not invited in. When you open your door, you are inviting specific people into the sacred space of your office. You say who is going to join and control the space as best you can.

For a virtual session on the phone or computer, you have a bit less control. You can certainly dictate when the session stops by monitoring when you allow the client onto the call. There is less that you can do about who shows up on the screen or where the client is. If you start a session and the client is either not in a place to do therapy or there are other people on the call that you did not expect, then you can most certainly ask for circumstances to change. You do not need to go ahead with virtual sessions if you cannot see the clients on the screen or they are not set up on their end to participate in the session.

When your in-person or telehealth session is almost up, you can send signals to the client that the session is nearly over. The end of the session is an important marker, as it creates a container for the work. When a client regularly violates that boundary, it can make the heart of the therapeutic work more challenging as it calls into question how deep to go and when to wrap up. If we know that we can touch into deeper emotions partway through the session and wrap up on time, then it allows us to safely move in and out of the deeper work. We do not want to go with the flow at the end of a session. Instead, it helps to have clearer boundaries at the end of sessions – unless a client brings up a traumatic event and you need to go with it for some time until it is properly closed up.

How you stop your sessions could reflect in some ways how you start your sessions. There are signals that we send the client when we start the conversation, encouraging them to get into the work. This mirrors signals that we send at the end of sessions suggesting that it is time to wrap up. For instance, do you do a lot of chit-chat at the beginning of a session? If so, then perhaps you move back into chit-chat at the end. Or do you start your sessions with a more direct question, such as "Where would you like to get started?" If the latter, it would be a good fit for you to be similarly direct about your session time coming to an end.

If you have a client who really will not stop at the end of sessions when you have sent the signals that time is up, then you might need to talk more explicitly about how you end sessions. For in-person sessions, you might also have to stand up from your chair, walk to the door and say farewell to get the client to stop. Virtual sessions often need a clear signal as well if the client pushes the boundary. If needed, you could stop your session a little early, knowing that you are going to have a longer goodbye process on the way out. One question you can ask yourself about any challenges to the end of session boundary is whether the client is aware that you are sending signals to end. Are they recognizing that the care and attention they were receiving during session are starting to fade? Are they aware that you are no longer as dialed in and that you want to wrap up?

Some of us can tell when the other person is not really listening or tuning in. But maybe for some clients, they are so used to not being heard that they keep going and going, and they do not read the feedback that you are done with the session. That could be something to talk about with them the next time you are in session.

One way of addressing it could be, "I feel like I do a better job of listening to you when we are sitting here, and I know last time we kept going past our time allotment. I am a little concerned that we did not address everything you wanted to talk about. I can't imagine you felt heard by me during that time."

The key is to keep your boundaries grounded in the relationship with the client. They should be mutually agreed upon, discussed, and be rooted in the spirit of care. One of the hardest things to be explicit about, and still express care, is to say no to a client. Telling them to stop, or even saying that you have to go to another meeting, can feel like a rejection for them. Being explicit about how you want to make boundaries while still expressing care is foundational to being effective as a clinician.

There are times to go with the flow and times to stop. In-session spontaneity must come to an end when the time is up. If all you did was go with the flow and be spontaneous, your sessions might not ever end. It would be too messy and chaotic. Yet if all you did was practice in an orderly and controlling manner, your work would be too clinical and cold. Chaos can be creative. You need both chaos and order to create healing. To make your session a balance of both chaos and order, you must find a way of gently reining in your spontaneity when it threatens to flow past the boundaries. Getting comfortable with containing, stopping, and saying no will not only help you, but it will also benefit the client.

5

ARE YOU A THERAPIST OR A PINEAPPLE? DON'T JUST DO SOMETHING, SIT THERE

In this chapter, we explore how active we should be in session. What do we do when a client talks the entire time? What about when they say very little? We explore how the basic process of therapy is that the client says something and we say something back. We are not just sitting there, we are doing something. Yet sometimes, it feels like if we do too much or say the wrong thing, we risk upsetting and triggering the client. Perhaps if we were just a pineapple sitting in the chair, not saying much, it would be safer! In this chapter, we discuss what to do when we let clients down and how the client understands their process with us.

Have something to say

Have you had clients talk with you about their experiences with previous therapists? It is usually a good approach to ask clients if they have been in therapy before just to get a general sense of their experience of the process. If they have seen other therapists before, you might want

DOI: 10.4324/9781003283164-6

to inquire as to what worked for them and also what did not. A client might respond with "Yeah, I saw this person. I don't even remember their name. It was okay."

That is not a very encouraging thing to hear! You might worry if they are going to remember your name. One major complaint that I hear is the perception that the previous therapist did not really say very much and that they just sat there. Hearing this might cause you to feel pressure to be more active in session than you normally would. We certainly want to hear what did not work for clients in previous therapy experiences and then try to correct it. If the complaint is that the previous therapist was not active enough, you have to find a way to have something to say.

Similarly, if the client shares something that has worked for them in past therapy experiences, then we will want to amplify that aspect of our work. If, for instance, they say that having concrete work to do between sessions really helped, then you will want to synthesize each session with some sort of homework. If you are less behavioral and more psychodynamic and the client says they want homework, then it is up to you to decide how much you are willing to adapt your work so that homework is provided. Perhaps you might take what they have learned in session and provide some bullet points for them to take home. Therapy is a co-created process between the therapist and the client, so we want to create something that will work for them. When a client says their past therapist did not do much and that they just sat there silently, then we must find a way to create a new experience for them.

One common factor across all modalities and theories of talk therapy is that the therapist talks. The client says something and the therapist says something back. Within that exchange, change and healing occur. It is better if what you say back has some substance and impact, but we ought to at least be ready to say something to the client so that there is some feedback happening for them. When you say "something" you at least contribute to the back and forth dialogue. It is better than saying nothing or uttering, "Hmm, okay, hmm, I see" all session long. That just leaves the client hanging there, waiting for you to interact. Perhaps you might ask them a question, and that will get some interaction going and allow you to think more clearly about how to intervene. At some point, the client is looking for more than just a series of questions. They eventually want you to take the information that you have gathered from listening to them and say something back to that has meaning and substance.

In this sense, a client is like a child with a bucket of Legos. What is the first thing the child will do with the bucket? They are going to pour all the Legos out on the ground. Similarly, when a client comes to session and dumps everything out by venting, they are simply expressing what has been happening in their lives. They want us to hear it. They also want us to do something with what we are hearing. They want us to help them put together what they are saying into something meaningful and useful. Just like with the Legos, we help them put the pieces together themselves so that they can make something useful out of what was spilled.

If a client started dumping a bunch of emotional Legos you would not just sit back and stay silent. Instead, you metaphorically might say, "Look, there is a blue Lego, there is a red one, there is a little Lego person." You piece a few items together and give it back to the client to see what they do with it. Engaging in this back and forth with what the client says keeps us out of being perceived as the do-nothing-say-nothing therapist who just sits there. We need to be prepared to say something, and to know that even just saying "something" back is curative.

Measuring therapy results

It is important to explain the process of therapy to the client so that they have a framework for how we are going to measure results. What people most complain about is that they did not see real, lasting change by participating in therapy. They put in a lot of time and effort, and did what the therapist asks of them, but they do not experience real results. Perhaps changes occur, but they are intangible and the client longs for more. Measuring change in therapy can be difficult. If you go to the hairdresser or barber, you may not like the haircut, but at least there are tangible results. With therapy, it is more subtle. We may need to help the client measure change and then talk about how we are tracking results.

Some people find it a relief when the therapist expresses their belief in the counseling process. The client wants to know that counseling works, and they want to feel the therapist's confidence in the process. They want to be in good hands with someone who can help them get to a better place and who also knows how to track the process. It can be useful, especially at the end of a first session, to summarize what took place and what the plan is moving forward.

For example, at the end of the first session, the therapist might say, "The first part of this meeting involved me gathering information from you, and in the middle I talked about some of the constraints to your happiness, how you sometimes do things that keep you from being happy. We started to look at some of the steps you could take to get rid of the patterns that made you unhappy. That is where we are at right now. Would you be open to seeing where we go from here?"

A lot of people think they know what therapy is like based on what they have seen on television or in the movies. They might not understand how you as the therapist work. You need to be constantly informing them of how you work and what your approach is. When you have breakthrough moments in session, or any "aha" experiences, it can help to comment on what happened for you and the client to get there. You become a narrator of the therapy process. You could say something like, "It took us many months of meeting to build trust and for us to develop this insight into your emotional patterns of relating. All of those sessions helped us get to this insight. This is how the process works. If I had said on the first day that your anger was connected to your low self-worth, it would not have had any impact and you would have rejected that interpretation. Or maybe you would have thought about it for a second but would not have had as deep an impact. All of our work has led to this understanding and it takes time."

Moments like this help the client see more keenly how therapy works. It can help cement the therapeutic relationship and create more of a buy-in to the therapy process. This usually happens somewhere in the middle of treatment. It is difficult to fully convey the process of therapy upfront, but perhaps you can suggest that you are going on a journey together with the client. They may have to actually experience the fact that real change takes time and that it occurs cumulatively, session after session.

Being patient in session

What do you do when your client does not agree with your interpretations? How do you handle it if they don't even let you get your complete observation out before they start negating what you have to say? It can be very demoralizing when a client asks for help but then rejects any suggestions you have. They might even compare you to a previous therapist who was "amazing" and so much more helpful, and it can leave you feeling ineffective. What do you do in those situations? It can be painful to feel like therapy is unproductive, but if you have patience, often something therapeutic will emerge.

In these instances, you may be surprised by how impactful it can be to simply be with the client. They get to talk and you listen to them. You might think that the session is not productive, but you could be wrong. Check with the client and ask them how the sessions are going from their perspective. They might report aspects of therapy helping them that you did not even realize were occurring. Perhaps you think nothing is happening, but the client is enjoying the conversation, and keeps returning week after week.

While you might be surprised that your clients keep coming back when sessions feel unproductive to you, something therapeutic could still be occurring for them. It can be challenging for the clinician, especially if you enjoy being more active in the room, to feel like not very much is happening in session, and that you are just like a pineapple sitting there doing nothing. You want to be active and make changes happen, yet when the therapy goes slowly, it can feel like you are not doing much more than sitting there.

In these instances, one thing to ask yourself is if you can be active, while also being patient. Your patience is your willingness to tolerate and sit with how this person is, how they cope, how they communicate. Your patience, week after week and month after month, might lead up to that one moment when a breakthrough occurs. All that waiting and listening becomes very much worth it when the "aha" moment happens. The answer to the question of what to do when they are talking, talking, talking and we feel like we're not being productive, is to be patient, knowing that something is happening there. We are at the very least thinking about the client and their development.

When the client is steamrolling us and keeps going and going without listening, we can shift toward working to understand what is happening. One thing that differentiates us from talking to a friend in a coffee shop is that we think about the other person in session. We think about their development, and we try to put their behavior into some sort of theoretical framework. We hypothesize about the case, knowing that we are patiently going somewhere. Pineapples cannot do any of that. Pineapples just sit there. Yet as a therapist who is present with the client, you are aware of what you are thinking about, even if it feels like you have to wade through a lot of data that the client shares in session. You might be surprised that your gentlest of touches in session can have a big impact on the client, even if you are simply being present with them.

When you try to help and the client rejects your offering, you can keep in mind that some of their rejection is simply a defense against receiving. It is a very vulnerable place to be on the receiving end of care, needing that care, and being open to taking it in. It is easier to give, as you are more in control when you are giving than when receiving. A way for the client to keep from being vulnerable is to either say nothing or fill the room with words, effectively rendering the therapist useless.

Most people experience their early caregivers or people in authority as ineffective. Clients will most likely perceive you as ineffective because it maps over their previous experiences of caregivers. It may not even matter what you do. You are likely going to get it wrong somehow and they are going to feel injured. Even though the client wants your help, they will do all sorts of things to keep you from being effective. They want you to be ineffective (at least the defensive part of them does), so they will experience you as ineffective, and you will experience yourself as ineffective. Yes, this is painful, especially for new clinicians, but what we want to do is keep going. We want to keep going and not get stuck there. We want to find a way to get through to the client even if at first they reject what we have to say.

You might need to pull out your bag of tricks to reach the highly defensive client. You could focus on partnering up with them in their struggles, or you could focus on witnessing the process of growth with them. They just need someone who is as developed as they are to be able to witness with them. There may be people in their lives who cannot appreciate all the nuances of who they are. But if you can stay with them, that can be all that the client needs. They have to really feel that you get them. You might say that one little thing that just synthesizes most of what they were saying in session, and that cements the therapeutic relationship because you met them in a way they have never been met before. With you, they might experience something that they usually never get: somebody who can actively hold space for them. You still have to do the talking and receiving because they need that. Yet your deep presence over time might be the curative factor.

Being humble

Bringing a deep sense of humility into session can help you meet the client where they are. The challenge we all face is in not knowing exactly what the client's mindset is when they come to session. One case example of this occurred for me a few years ago where a male individual in his 40s came in and was telling me about a horrible experience with his father, who left him when he was young. He recounted how his stepfather came into the picture, and after he became close with his stepfather, he left his mother when the client was 12. It was a horrible injury and really impacted the client terribly. He told me all of this within the first 20 minutes of the first session. In response to him saying that it impacted him terribly, I asked, "in what ways?" And he said indignantly, "In what ways? I just told you all this stuff about my father leaving me, and then my stepfather leaving me, and you coldly ask me, 'in what ways?'" He stood up, came toward me, and put out his hand to shake mine and said, "This clearly is not going to work." He put the intake paperwork on my desk and left.

I remember sitting there, looking out the window for another 20 minutes, wondering what happened. What did I just do? How did I get this so wrong? I took it to supervision, and we came up with a plan that I should call him and apologize.

> I called him and said, "I know that session didn't feel very good."
> He said, "Yeah, it did not feel good. I came in looking for help."
> "That must have felt horrible," I replied. "Maybe I could set you up with a colleague who could be more helpful than I was."

He agreed and took the referral. I gave a hard look at what I did wrong, and I could not find very much. I had not even started any sort of intervention. I greeted him warmly, but maybe not warmly enough. I listened but maybe not actively enough. I determined that he was spring-loaded, ready to be disappointed and let down. I did not understand why things became so reactive such that he left, but I think the thing about people being disappointed is that when we let them down, we need to be prepared for how they are going to cope with that.

I would hope a client like this, when I asked, "in what ways," would say something like "Well, it's kind of obvious how it impacted me, but I'd be happy to tell you. But in fact, your question 'in what ways' makes me feel like you don't get it and that you're not listening." Yet that is not realistic. Instead, what is more typical is that the client plays out their disappointments and wounds with us. This first session was likely an enactment of the client being wounded previously. It may not have mattered what I did. I was set up to be the disappointing or neglectful caregiver. There was likely a parataxic distortion occurring in which I was not seen clearly. I need to understand that I am being experienced through the lens of previous helpers.

When a client's perspective of us is distorted like this, such that it does not even matter what we say, it can feel unfair to the therapist. When the client says that their previous therapist was horrible, and that they just sat there, we can take it with a grain of salt because that could have been us just sitting there, experienced by the client through a distorted lens. The client might experience something we said or did wrong, or didn't do at all, and see us as ineffective. We are human and often do not get it right. Yet who knows how the client takes us in? This client from my past might have talked with the new therapist and said, "I went to this therapist and he said it was all about my father, and it made no sense. He didn't care, I would never go back there again. When I told him about my past, all he could say was 'in what ways.' He was a horrible therapist."

He may very well have experienced me in this negative light, which is not easy to tolerate as a therapist who cares about the client experience. When we are not given a chance to help but also handle such an extreme distortion of perception based on the client's experiences, it can be quite painful and humbling. To get through it, I must first start to see that he must be really hurting. I need to feel safe enough to generate this sort of compassion. If I feel safe enough within myself, then I have a chance to go into that humble space where I can see how opening up in therapy must have been hard for this client.

It is also a real challenge for the therapist when we do not feel secure in session and have clients' distorted transferences coming at us. Our guard is down, and we have to contain the full range of the client's distress and potential acting out. When they are disappointed in us and the stakes are high, it can be tempting to just sit there like a pineapple and not say anything harmful. At least being a pineapple is harmless for the most part. It is not doing anything that is going to elicit any kind of hurt. Yet if you are active and try to do something, you risk being experienced as neglectful or hurtful. We can wonder if it would be better to sit there as pineapples because at least we aren't risking saying the wrong thing.

There is a lot to learn from these sorts of situations. Without getting ourselves too freaked out, we need to remind ourselves that people are vulnerable when they come in to meet with us. We do not know what mental state they are in when they enter the room. They might be spring-loaded emotionally or vulnerable to being triggered by a disappointing caregiver. They expect a lot from us and for the most part, we find a way to reach them. But when we get it wrong, we need to find a way to adapt. If we are given the chance to say "oh, I really hurt you there. I'm sorry," we have a chance to meet the client on a compassionate level. By softening our approach, we might be better received and be able to communicate more directly. The experience of getting it wrong as the therapist is baked in. You cannot overcome it. It is part of the process of trying to help people. Yet your willingness to still try to say something that will help can make a big difference in the client's life.

6

WHEN YOUR CLIENT GHOSTS YOU: HOW TO KEEP CLIENTS

This chapter focuses on how to manage clients when they stop coming to therapy without communicating with us. Do we chase them down for a termination session? Do we let them go? Should we hold a spot for them in our caseload if they canceled the last few weeks? What do you do when a client ghosts you and just stops coming to therapy? The chapter explores ways to manage one's caseload.

Dealing with ghosts

What do you do when it's uncertain whether or not a client will engage in therapy with you? What do you do when they just fade from the process a little bit and do not schedule follow-up sessions? Often the harbinger of a client terminating might be last-minute cancellations, a lot of schedule changes, or the client regularly saying that they cannot make it to session. This may be a signal that therapy is winding down. It is important to keep in mind that therapy stopping may not always

DOI: 10.4324/9781003283164-7

correlate with treatment being concluded. There might be more work to be done, yet for various reasons, the client might stop therapy. A client wanting to reduce the regularity of their attendance can indicate that their commitment to therapy is waning.

Back in the early days of psychoanalysis, if the client would say, "I want to stop therapy," the analyst would interpret it as resistance and insist that the treatment continue. Today we work collaboratively. We co-create the therapy process with the client. If they start to exhibit signs of wanting to stop therapy while we think there is a lot of work to do to resolve the presenting issues, we can recommend that therapy continue. Yet that does not necessarily mean that the client is going to take our advice.

I once had a college-aged client reengage for a session while she was home from school over winter break. I anticipated that we would talk about her development, how she was managing her ongoing depression, and how school was going this semester. Yet when we talked, she simply wanted to focus on if she should send her ex-boyfriend a card for his birthday. Even though I thought there was a lot of developmental and adjustment work to be done, she just wanted to focus on how to handle her ex-boyfriend's birthday. While I thought it would help to discuss other topics, the client benefitted more from talking about the ex-boyfriend's birthday. It helped when I met the client where she was rather than forwarding my agenda.

Clients come to therapy for all sorts of reasons, and it may be very different from why you think they are there. As much as we want the course of treatment to follow what we think should happen, it might not. When it veers off-course from our expectations, just like my session with the student home from college, it can feel chaotic. We may question our ability to know what are we even doing.

I have supervised therapists who work in a college drop-in center where it is not necessarily long-term therapy. In those situations, it is difficult to predict what the course of therapy might be. Students would often come in with what the faculty identified as a crisis because of emotional meltdowns in class. When they showed up, we could not predict how long therapeutic engagement would be, so we tried to clean up any mess from the presenting crisis and create a format for potential engagement in long-term therapy. We had to work within the unpredictable structure of a drop-in center and try our best to be supportive while the student was there.

In private practice, we can feel like we have more control over the structure than if we work in a school or other setting where the structure may be dictated by external forces. Yet there are still a lot of unknowns wherever we practice, and it helps if we adjust our protocols so that they are fluid and ready for uncertainty. If you have a client that you see the first time on Wednesday at 4 o'clock in the afternoon, they may not necessarily be your Wednesday 4 o'clock client each week. We do not know how long the client is going to stay engaged and even if the 4 o'clock time slot will work for them going forward. As much as you might want to have control over your schedule, it is more helpful to stay open to clients moving fluidly in and out of different time slots. Being flexible often helps with keeping balance in your caseload. Clients may stop coming to therapy but then resume a few months later once they are feeling overwhelmed again. Accounting for these sorts of uncertainties allows you to fit more clients into your weekly schedule.

Of course, having some clear boundaries helps. For instance, if there is a higher risk case and the client stops coming to therapy, then we would want to close their file rather than leave the case open should they want to return later. We want there to be a hard demarcation about in-treatment and out-of-treatment in those situations. If there is a risk of suicidality, homicidality, or if the person has higher-level emotional issues, then we want to have a clear point of stopping treatment with them. You can send a letter or an email documenting that you have not heard from the client in awhile and that you are going to take that as communication that they no longer interested in continuing treatment. You should be clear that you are closing their file, and if at any point they want to reengage, they can let you know, and you would be happy to open their file again. In this instance, you are indicating that the file is closed, protecting you from liability. In your message, you can convey that by saying, "I am going to close your file. Should you ever want to reengage, I cannot promise you our same time slot, or that I will have immediate openings, but I would be happy to try to get you back in to see me."

For the most part, we want to try to get clients that we have seen before back in to see us again. This can create challenges in balancing our caseload when we try to fit old clients back in among our current and newer cases. If, for instance, your caseload is pretty full, and a client you have seen every week for two years stops for the summer but wants to come back in once the summer ends, you may really want to try to find a way to get them back on your schedule. Other than with high-risk cases, you can choose how you want to communicate with clients who stop regularly coming to session. You can always contact them about coming back in, but they will usually communicate with their feet. They either keep coming in or they just don't show up, and then you know they have stopped.

The more confident you are in your work, the less anxious you will feel about clients returning to you or not. If they are not coming back, it is either because they are not ready to do the work or it was not a fit for them to work with you, and they found somebody else. Often clients will give up on the therapy process and do not feel comfortable having a conversation with you in person, letting you know that it is not working for them. They fear telling you that it is not helping. Many high-functioning clients, when asked about their negative therapy experience, say they fear talking with their counselor about their dissatisfaction. They worry that the therapist will take it personally or that the therapist will not be there to help them should the client want to return. If the client has their own issues around authority and caregivers, then they may shy away from talking with you about why they want to stop treatment. Instead, they just won't show up to the next session.

Handling sudden termination

When a client suddenly terminates by not showing up, it can help if you invite them in for a termination session. It can sometimes bear fruit and they will reengage. However, often they won't respond, and you won't hear from them again. In those cases, it can feel like the request for a termination session is more for you than for them. If you word your request in a way, either voicemail or email, your message to them might allow them a chance to get back into therapy with you.

You can say something like, "I know we have not been meeting regularly lately, and I think it would be useful for us to do one more meeting as a closing session to wrap up and terminate our work. Let me know if you would be up for that." Typically, you should charge for that termination session, but if it seems appropriate, you can say you would be happy to not charge them for the meeting because you think it would be really useful to talk.

If you saw the client for at least eight to ten sessions, then reaching out for a termination session is appropriate. If you only had a few weeks of therapy with them, then there often is not very much to wrap up. The client just might not feel that it was a fit for them, and they do not feel comfortable talking with you about it.

Sometimes during that termination session, the client reengages in therapy and the work resumes. They talk about why they stopped coming but then start discussing what else is going on in their lives. They find the session helpful and want to get back to seeing you regularly. In those cases, it has been worth it to do that termination session, even if it was complimentary because now the client has reengaged in therapy. You could offer a wrap-up session to see if they will communicate with you.

There is so much uncertainty in these sorts of situations. I remember telling my supervisor when I was in training that a client was complaining that the therapy with me was not helping them. My supervisor said that was a good sign that they were telling me.

I was confused. Why is it a good thing that a client is telling me that therapy wasn't working? Shouldn't I be concerned that they are unhappy?

He asked me whether I would rather have my clients tell me that therapy is not working for them or have them not say anything at all. His stance was that he would want to know if a client is unhappy. He would want to hear from them what is not working or what is not feeling right so that he might be able to fix it. He would want to invite the client to tell him if something did not feel right about therapy. He even included this as an expectation at the beginning of treatment while also inviting regular progress check-ins throughout the course of treatment.

Being ghosted by clients

Even with a clear expectation about checking in about the process of treatment, the concern is that for the most part, clients probably will not tell us what isn't working for them in the therapy. They often just leave. They ghost us. We never hear from them again. In those instances, you are left to do your own reflection about what went wrong. Perhaps it was when you changed the meeting time that the rupture in the therapeutic relationship happened. Or perhaps the way you communicated that change of time came across as if the client was not important to you. You can at least do an assessment, either in consultation or on your own, about what went wrong. You can try to identify everything you can, but there are some things you just won't know. Sometimes you won't have more information about why the client is not coming back, and you never get that kind of closure. Those are humbling moments.

It is very unsatisfying when there is not any sort of closure. Even our most favorite clients may ghost us and not return to therapy ever again, without any communication. We can have deep, close, satisfying relationships with clients that end without notice. We need to be prepared for that. Clients might just slip away at any point.

I have had clients ghost me a number of times. One wrote me recently after slipping away two years prior, saying, "Well that was a long pause. I've had a lot going on but I would like to come back to therapy." Two years felt like more time to me than a long pause! I replied that I would love to see him again and asked when he would like to meet. Yet he never replied to that message and ultimately did not come back in, even with a follow-up message on my part. I do not know what happened and why he reached out but failed to follow through with scheduling a session. I must have represented something to him enough that he thought about me and reached out in a moment of need. As his therapist, I am somebody who is in his corner and am there for him when he needs help. He might still be ambivalent about working with me and may continue to slip in and out of therapy for years. If a client slips away, there is always a possibility they might reemerge out of nowhere only to leave us again. We need to be prepared for that too.

We also do not need to chase clients down or check in with them repeatedly. It is not like they forgot about therapy, and then we remind them, and they say to themselves, "Oh yeah, I should go into therapy." They know we are there. They know they can reach out, and we will welcome them in. Our role is to be a good attachment object, somebody who is holding space but not pressuring them. Clients will come in when they are ready. If they need to spin out and go away for a while, that is fine. When they are ready to engage, they will come in.

With that approach, being open to clients coming and going as they need to, your caseload may be a lot bigger than your current, active roster. You may have a bullpen of other clients who can always come back to you at any time. It feels good to be that sort of force for people in their lives that should they ever want to return, you will be there. The challenge is how to get them back into your schedule when they return. You might even have to put them on a waiting list. The key is to try to be there for returning clients because normally, they do not want to get started with anyone else. They need a person they know they can depend on who is there for them in the long run.

Structuring schedules and caseloads

To create balance, you can consider adopting a more fluid schedule. This starts with structuring the course of treatment so that it begins in a measured way. One option is to do a number of allotted sessions and assess the client's progress after those sessions. At that point, you could add another block of sessions and assess from there. Alternatively, you could work on the presenting issue until both you and the client have a sense that it has been resolved. At that point, you then reassess the goals of therapy and what the structure of it will be. This approach is more of a solution-focused one where you focus on the work that is part of the presenting problem and then consult on how and why you might continue.

One reason not to have too many clients on your caseload is that you may not realistically be able to be there for 40–50 people should they all want to see you weekly. Sometimes it may be advisable to have fewer clients and see them each weekly. Other times, it works to see them every other week. It all depends on the presenting problem and symptoms.

Your schedule can include some regular weekly clients who you see at the same time each week while also having others who you piece into your schedule week-to-week, at various times. Perhaps you might have half of your schedule be regular appointments and the other half be room for people to float in and out. You can place more people on your caseload if they have flexible schedules.

If you have a lot of clients whose schedules are not flexible, then you might need to get creative. Can you work with them to find times that fit for their schedule that also work with your availability? It can feel awful when clients are on breaks or move to an every-other-week schedule, and you can't fill the alternate weeks or open time slot. You are left sitting there in an empty office having lost an hour in your caseload. In this case, it can be helpful to have more flexibility and place someone into the open time slot. Being excessively rigid with your schedule will not allow for this. While it might give you some comfort to have a sense of control or regularity, it can backfire when you have too many open holes in your schedule.

Having a more fluid schedule errs on the side that you can see more people on a more consistent basis, even if they are flowing in and out of various time slots. Your caseload actually ends up being more full because you can provide more fluid scheduling options. Whereas if you are more rigid with your schedule, you might end up saying, "No, I can't see you," or "No, I can't take that case," more often than you would like. To create a more fluid schedule, you would not hold specific time slots for clients. Instead, you would schedule them week to week. At the end of each session, you would ask when they want to meet next. While keeping your hours of availability regular, you would work with the client to determine the frequency and timing of meetings.

When your schedule is full, you may be full for a little while. A caseload in private practice is kind of an organic being, where it goes from full to empty and then back to full pretty quickly. There are certain times of the year, for example, when clients return after the summer break, that might be busier than other times when it is slower. You will also need to let go of old ways of scheduling if they start to work against you. Some people like working only three or four long days a week. They enjoy their days off, but then they realize those long clinical days are horrible, so they change their schedule. You can change it up too.

7

CARING FOR YOUR CLIENTS WHILE TAKING NOTES

This chapter looks the administrative aspects of being a clinician and how it is the key to being successful as a therapist. Many of us separate the administrative aspects of our work from caring for our clients, yet it could be one of the more important things that we do for them. Progress notes, treatment summaries, billing reports, and emails from clients ... all of it goes into the care that we give. Being vigilant about how we operate administratively can go a long way toward serving our clients more fully. Topics include how to attend to the financial and insurance aspects of our work and how caring for our clients is intimately tied to administrative and business tasks.

How to take a note when you're exhausted

It may be the end of a long day seeing clients and responding to emails, and the last thing that a weary therapist wants to do is write their clinical notes. If they have seen just a few clients, or especially if they have had a full day of back-to-back sessions, it can feel arduous to have to

DOI: 10.4324/9781003283164-8

document the day's work. Many therapists report telling themselves that they will do the note later when they get home from the office. Others promise that they will do all of their notes at the end of the week. Some make time between sessions or at the end of the day at the office to do their notes. Regardless of the routine, note-taking is an essential part of caring for our clients and should be seen as an extension of the session, not something separate.

For a lot of eager therapists, the clinical hour is the most enjoyable and energizing part of the work. Getting more connected with the client, making discoveries, finding insights, and opening new perspectives can connect us to the sacredness of what we feel called to do as a livelihood. We dream of making a deep impact in people's lives and often can remember key cases in our training that helped form what we knew could be possible in therapy. Most of us don't dream of case notes, treatment plans, and treatment summaries. We are taught that it is an important task and essential to best practices, yet clinical paperwork often does not inspire lofty ideation.

To many clinicians, case notes, billing, and administrative work are a means to an end. They are the necessary evils that we must endure in order to practice the craft that we love. This in-session love version out-of-session administrative tedium can set up the modem therapist to become weary of paperwork and neglect this essential piece of professional functioning. If we love what we do when we are sitting in our therapist chair, but feel like we must endure the tasks associated with sitting at our desk, then we miss an opportunity to find meaning in all aspects of being a clinician. Worse yet, we create an imbalance as we move from therapist chair to desk and back again.

The pull of two chairs

Many times over the course of my career, I have found myself sitting at my office desk working on an email, treatment plan, or session note, only to find that it is the top of the hour and that my next client is in the waiting room. I might still need to run to the bathroom, make a cup of tea, or attend to something happening in my personal life. It becomes a crunch for time. Perhaps you have found yourself if this sort of situation as well. There is a tension when you wish you could be sitting at your desk, working on your emails, notes, or personal projects, but in order to start the next session on time, you find yourself sitting in your therapist chair saying hello to the next client, wishing that you were still at your desk.

I am ashamed to admit that I have started many sessions with my body in my therapist chair, but my mind still wandering over to the desk and the administrative work that I did not fully finish. My shame comes from acting as if I was present with the client while, in all honesty, I was still thinking about the note that needed to be finished or the email I was in the middle of composing. In those moments, it likely seemed to the client that I was listening to them, but my attention was really elsewhere, wishing that I had more time at my desk to complete the administrative tasks that were on my to-do list.

Because I pride myself on being present with my clients, it feels especially unpleasant, imbalanced, and downright inauthentic to be caught in the tension between the therapy chair and the desk chair. The back and forth tends to cause me more stress than it should, and I have had to find ways to carve out more time for the business of being a therapist. When I use my between-session time to instead take care of and nourish myself, I tend to feel less stressed in session. My attention and presence are more dialed in on the contents of the beginning of session. Problems arise when I catch sight of emails or calls from clients during those few minutes between sessions. I have to be disciplined not to check my email or get pulled into an administrative task. Rather, it has been more helpful when I set aside separate time each day to care for the administrative elements associated with my work.

The joy of to-do lists

The process of therapy is ongoing and unfolding. Seldom are we able to cross an item off a list of therapeutic goals for the client. It is not as if we are able to complete or solve the task of eliminating their anxiety, for example. Therapy is not that easy to measure. It is more gradual, and we need to be patient. Yet, with administrative work, we do get to have a sense of completion. We write that note or send that email. Our to-do list can be completed, and that can be a nice counterbalance to the ambiguous nature of pursuing therapy goals.

We can also feel pulled to focus more and more on administrative work because it provides us with a sense of accomplishment. We might want to spend more time at our desks taking care of emails, notes, and plans than sitting in session with clients. The satisfaction of checking items off of our to-do lists can be alluring compared to the constant uncertainty of clinical work. It would be very normal if you enjoy the accomplishment that comes with business items or administrative tasks. Those activities can give us a more instant sense of competency. Therapy, on the other hand, will constantly teach us that there is much to learn and that we are far from mastering our craft.

We just want to be careful not to become overly absorbed in business tasks. There can be a workaholism associated with obsessively focusing on billing, accounts receivable, or emails instead of attending more meaningfully to our clients. If we avoid the uncomfortable uncertainty of helping other human beings in favor of more defined administrative tasks, then we lose sight of the heart of our work. We forget that our caring presence is the most valuable tool that we have. Our ability to check insurance claims is important, but it is not at the core of what we do. Nor is it at the core of who we are. As instruments of our craft, who we are informs the work we do. Sitting with clients, thinking through their presenting problems, and creating opportunities for new insights is a creative expression of who you are. It is the work of putting your own healing and personal growth into the service of others. While we might get caught up in all the administrative tasks that come with being a clinician, we must not lose sight of the core of what we do.

Business structure

We also need to be careful not to neglect our administrative lives. If we feel so pulled by the artistic expression of being a therapist in session that we let our notes and emails slip away, then we neglect the framework that holds the therapeutic process together. We are required to document our sessions, and we owe it to our clients to be on top of scheduling, billing, and communication. We cannot be successful clinicians without being stellar administrators. Too many clinicians imagine that they will have someone else handle all the business tasks for them while they get to focus solely on clinical work. This is possible in some situations, but I think that it is important that we are competent with all aspects of our practice. If we take responsibility for billing, scheduling, notes, payment for sessions, and communication with clients, then it provides a sort of wraparound, comprehensive care that comes through in the clinical work.

I know of a number of talented clinicians who bring so much skill to the clinical work but who have neglected the administrative aspects of their practice. While their presence in session is terrific, and their creativity with clients is transformative, their oftentimes willful neglect of the business side of therapy has caused their practices to fall apart. For example, clinicians who fail to submit insurance claims on time, leaving enormous deductible payments to pile up for clients, can cause the client to have to flee from therapy because they owe hundreds of dollars and are unable to pay. If the therapeutic alliance had grown and the client had become hopeful about therapeutic progress, but billing insurance claims and handling the financial aspects of treatment are mismanaged, then treatment of the client will likely fall apart. In this case, if we checked benefits or submitted a claim at the first session to see what the coverage is and then communicated that information to a client, it would build a better framework for therapy so that the work is sustainable.

The business side of practicing holds therapy together. It creates the groundwork for meaningful treatment to occur. Many new clinicians are so enamored by the intimacy that comes with working with clients in session that they fail to learn the ins and outs of the business side of our work. They let supervisors, admin staff, or insurance billers take care of the back-end tasks rather than learning these tasks themselves. This leaves gaping holes in their competency as clinicians and sets them up for more colossal failures that can let clients down. Not documenting sessions on time, not submitting claims to insurance, making mistakes billing the client appropriately, or mismanaging your schedule can cause all the good clinical work to go out the window. The client will end up feeling neglected should you fail to manage finances, insurance, or scheduling well. If you are not comfortable with billing, scheduling, submitting insurance, claims, taking notes, or communicating with your clients between sessions, then it would help to work on those items in supervision so that you are prepared to hold clients more substantively.

Careful notes

A clinical note is also part of holding clients. While we learn in graduate school the basics of documenting sessions, we often do not connect the important process of taking notes to the care that we offer our clients. Instead, we often see it as a side task that needs to be done for HIPAA compliance. We relegate note-taking to the mundane red tape that comes with bureaucracy, or we do the note because our supervisors will be reading them.

Some new clinicians will spend too much time on their notes, writing out everything that they do in sessions so that their supervisor will have a sense of what is occurring. These novellas that are written by new therapists go into too much detail about the session and take too much time to write. If you cannot write a typical clinical note in one to two minutes, then you are likely writing too much. Unless there is a risk item involved in the case, a common clinical note should be a distillation of the interventions that you used in session. It should document and illuminate the heart of the work that you are doing. Being able to succinctly communicate in the client's record the care that you are providing is an essential aspect of being a therapist. The key is to be able to effectively name the presenting problem and your intervention. Instead of writing a detailed account of the conversation in therapy, we need to summarize it in a sentence or two.

For instance, if an individual client was talking in session about struggles with their former spouse, how the holidays create tension with co-parenting, and how they are wrestling with what they should do about going to their new romantic partner's holiday family gathering, then you do not need to write out all of the details in your note. Instead, it helps to find a way to name the theme that is behind all of this content. You have to read between the lines and connect with what the client is wrestling with beneath all of the details. In this case, your note might describe the presenting issue as "boundary management in intimate relationships" or "navigating new patterns of relating." However you describe it, if you can distill the contents down to the core themes that present in therapy, then you do yourself a favor by shortening the time it takes to write the note. You also do the client a big favor because it also helps you get clear about what you are working on with them in treatment.

For the above example, if you intervene by asking the client about how they remember their divorced parents navigating the holiday season, then your note might read, "Connected to family of origin patterns." If you intervene by encouraging them to talk with each person about their needs for the holidays, then you might document the intervention as, "Worked on effective means of communication." You might also include any models of therapy that you use such as "Used Cognitive Behavioral Therapy to help client create clear boundaries."

Your note will most certainly be dictated by the context in which you are working. You would have to abide by the requirements of your place of practice and any supervisory oversight. Yet the key is to find a way to infuse your clinical notes with care and make them a clear expression of the important work you are doing without it taking too much time. Connecting the love you provide in session with sound business practices can create a solid foundation for your clients to feel fully supported.

8

THE INS AND OUTS OF TRANSFERENCE

This chapter discusses how to work with transference and countertransference and what happens when we try to shift those transferences. We also discuss what to do when the transference from our client makes us feel good versus when it makes us uncomfortable, as well as when to take risks to challenge our clients within the therapeutic relationship.

Transference and countertransference

What is transference, and how do we work with it so that it serves the client? One definition of transference is the redirection of unconscious material from one object to another.[1] From an object-relations perspective, an object would be a person who has been significant to the client. The client unconsciously takes some of the feelings, thoughts, and reactions they have toward that person, and they transfer it to someone else, in this case, the therapist. Freud called transference an acting out

DOI: 10.4324/9781003283164-9

of unconscious fantasies as a defense against remembering.[2] Instead of remembering and resolving what happened in our lives, we keep playing out aspects of it and transferring it onto somebody else. We take our reactions to an important person in our lives and project them onto the other person. When a client does this to the therapist, it is called transference. Countertransference is the therapist's redirection of unconscious material from other things or people in their life back onto the client. The client could remind you of a sibling, for instance, or a previous partner, and you might have reactions to the client that are similar to how you reacted to that other person in your life.

These phenomena are all pretty normal, and we would be wise to work with them and be conscious of them. We do not necessarily want to throw off the transference from our client when it is coming at us. We want to make use of it for the therapeutic process. If, for instance, the client says something like "You are so brilliant" or "You seem to always have the answers," you do not necessarily need to throw off the compliment and act demurely. You also do not need to cultivate the qualities or persona of that transference. Instead, you might say thank you and then admit that certainly, you do not have all the answers but that you are trying your best to help the client find a resolution to their issues. If the client feels like they are in competent hands with you, even if it is part of their transference, you might be able to work with that to help them make progress more quickly in therapy.

You want to work with whatever the client is sending toward you about how they are experiencing you. Doing so helps unlock how they relate to others or what gets in their way of feeling more connected to themselves or the world. You might handle all sorts of transferences, and they might span a wide range. For example, a client may have an erotic transference toward you and feel an attraction. That can be very uncomfortable to be on the receiving end of it, and it would make sense that you would want to throw that off of you. You would also ethically need to be clear about the therapeutic relationship and that it does not involve social or romantic interaction. Simultaneously, you might also be able to work with this sort of transference in some instances. You could ask yourself what it is about what you are doing or representing to the client that is making them feel connected or close to you. You will also want to know why the connection is becoming eroticized while being sure to adhere to professional standards of care. Maybe the client is experiencing you as someone who cares about them, and they confuse care with physical attraction. If it feels comfortable, you could explore that with them in a way that helps the therapeutic process. Whatever you do, in general, we want to make sure the ethical boundaries are made explicit while working with the transferences that come our way rather than ignoring them.

Working with clients' transferences

What if a client gets stuck in their projection and does not ever see us clearly for who we are? This can be a frustrating experience for the therapist. Even if we try to reveal who we are to the client, they still might keep pulling us back into their projections. These situations could be called parataxic distortions in which the client skews their perception of you so much that it stays in fantasy, and they never see you clearly. The term parataxic distortion comes from psychoanalyst Harry Stack Sullivan and is derived from a Greek term meaning "placement side by side." The prefix "para" suggests a derivative from the base word (like *para*normal). "Taxic" in this case, indicates movement toward or away from a specific stimulus. So parataxic distortion would be a shift in perception away from reality.[3]

It is safe to assume that pretty much every client who experiences us will have a parataxic distortion of us. They will not see us clearly – nor do we need them to. They experience us through various lenses, such as an authority or parental figure, for better or for worse. This can happen in the blink of an eye, as the client will come up with an assumption about who we are based on the first interaction, or perhaps even sooner – when they are first referred to us. We do not need to be overly invested in the client accurately seeing us for who we are because no matter what we do, they certainly may not see us clearly. Instead, we want to understand what sort of distortions they are having in order to figure out how that impacts them and the therapeutic relationship. If the distortion is so strong that good therapy cannot occur, then we must work to throw the distortion off as best we can.

For example, an inexact interpretation can help in instances when the client sees us as the all-knowing authority. We could resist the urge to have the answers to their questions and instead encourage them to find meaning and clarify their thinking. Or, if there is a maternal or paternal transference, perhaps you can say something that challenges the transference so that they are forced to take you in as a full person. From a humanistic approach to counseling, the therapist-client relationship is central, and you want to have the client grapple with taking you in as a full person. We do not want to leave them with just their distortions or projections of us. We want them to incorporate other data about who we are so that the care and support they experience in therapy can be more easily exported into other relationships in their life. This shift of moving the transference into something more human is essential to how the therapeutic relationship can create healing. Being able to do this takes practice and training.

First, you have to *notice* when you are on the receiving end of transference or a projection. After you have seen enough clients to know what you normally feel when you are working in session, you will have a sense of when you are on the receiving end of a projection because you will start to feel and think differently than normal. After you have enough therapy hours under your belt, you will notice a basic range of thoughts and feelings you normally have as a clinician. When your thoughts and feelings start going way outside of that range, then that is probably a good indication that you are on the receiving end of a projection.

If you find yourself ruminating about a case or taking it home with you, you might be experiencing client transference as well. Clients' projections can fill us up emotionally and cause us to feel more stirred than usual. This further intensifies when we identify with their projection and introject it into ourselves. This is called projective identification. For example, if the client says, "You seem like a great mother," you might identify with that and think, "Yes, I am a great mother. I can take care of this person." This might feel good in the moment, but when you are overly invested and thinking about the client too often outside of session, then it can cause a problem for the relationship.

Even if you do not identify and internalize the projection, when you notice it coming at you, the next step is to disturb the transference in some way. You might move, upset or shift the transference so that it does not stay static. Changing the way the client actually experiences you so that their transference on you changes can be done in a healthy way and align with the therapeutic goal. For example, if the goal is for the client to become more empowered in their life and trust their own ability to make decisions, maybe we do not want to foster an idealized transference onto the therapist as somebody who has all the answers. If the client has an idealized transference, then we want to transition the transference into something else other than as an expert so that it does not keep invalidating the client's experience. In this situation, in order to avoid dependency, we could shift the transference from all-knowing sage to someone who cares about them yet may not have all the answers. This, in turn, allows the client to access their own wisdom.

Transitioning the transference in this way would be taking a risk because it would upset the apple cart. There is a sort of agreement between you and the client that you are going to be open to receive whatever way the client experiences you. In other words, they expect you to be open to their transferences. While it might feel safer to keep with this agreement and stay within the client's distortions of you because it keeps the therapeutic relationship stable, we best serve the therapeutic work by throwing off the transference. If you disrupt or challenge the transference, then it allows the therapeutic process to go further. Even if it is unsettling for the client to be disillusioned, it is often done for the greater good.

Defending against positive transference

Beware of positive transference because there is always a flip side. If you are experienced by the client as a positive force, perhaps a validating mother or father figure, then they might also have a conversely negative experience of you as a scolding mother or a punitive, withholding father. If you experience excessive positive transference from a client, you might need to draw a boundary at some point in order to protect against the flip side of the transference, which might come your way if you ever let them down. Should you ever be out of town when the client needs you most, or if you get something wrong in session, or if you challenge the client a bit too hard, then they might not just feel let down professionally – they might also experience that disappointment through a distorted lens and see a de-idealized mother or father figure.

Knowing that there is a flip side coming whenever you feel positive transference will help you not identify too much with it. You can instead understand how the client experiences care and support and help the entire therapy process stay grounded in the moment. Your goal is to have a more present exchange where the client is able to see you clearly, with a little bit less distortion. You are not the mother, you are not a guru, you are not saving them. You are helping them gain insight into themselves so they can heal and make the changes that they need.

From countertransference to intervention

A neutral stance of unconditional positive regard goes a long way when navigating confusing transferences with clients. When considering our own countertransference, we could look more deeply at what unconditional positive regard really means. It is not realistic to meet every presenting problem with unconditional positive regard. You might have judgments about some of the unhealthy behaviors of your clients. If on some level, you are judging your client yet you try to take an unconditionally positive stance, then there is something inauthentic happening. It does not serve the client for you to feel one way about them and act another. If the therapist cannot be genuine with their client, then who can? We must try to find a way to turn our reactions into interventions rather than burying what we feel.

To do this, we have to get a handle on what our reactions are to our clients presenting issues and work through our countertransference. Consultation and supervision are important places where we can talk through our reactions. Our own individual therapy can be a place to unpack what we bring to our sessions as well. We certainly do not want to have our reactions and judgments come spilling out raw in session. That could be demeaning and is unprofessional. We also do not want to push away our countertransference and bury it. Instead, we ought to work with countertransference and then turn it into an intervention that will serve the client.

Suppose a male client discloses to you that he has been fantasizing about female coworkers and has been making inappropriate passes at them. You likely would have a negative reaction. If you tried to keep up an unconditional positive regard in this situation and pretended to be understanding, it would ring false, and you would be tacitly condoning his behavior. If you scolded him and told him that his behavior is not okay and that it is likely hurting people and making them uncomfortable, you risk shaming him and compromising the therapeutic relationship. The goal would be to try to take your reactions, get a consultation if needed, and turn them into an effective intervention. Your goal might eventually be to understand why he is acting inappropriately and work toward finding compassion for him while not condoning his unhealthy behavior.

Perhaps in this sort of situation, you could say, "You matter, but not to these women at work, and not in that way. I see how badly you want and need to matter, and to matter to certain people in certain ways. What if a coworker thought you mattered but not in a sexual way? Is there something about getting attention from women that makes you matter?"

Sex is very validating, so maybe you can challenge the client in a way that is palatable. "We have been meeting for a number of sessions now, and I think what you are talking about is very important. I would like to see you feel fulfilled. Yet I'm worried that you are just getting a substitute for fulfillment by hitting on your coworkers and fantasizing about them. This is not the real nourishment of life that is going to help you feel truly alive. It is more like being addicted to junk food. You can eat and it feeds you, but ultimately it's not very nourishing or healthy. I want you to experience very satisfying interactions that are make you feel like you matter."

The key is to work with your reactivity to clients like this, understand your judgment, and find ways to process them so that they turn into effective interventions. The negative feelings that you have about your clients may not be judgments, they might just be negative feelings. You don't have to positively regard everything that a client says. You can maintain your congenial relationship with the client and still have a mixture of feelings in response to what they are presenting. It would be weird to respond positively when a client expresses something disturbing. When a client says something shocking, it would be more genuine to be shocked than to remain cool or dispassionate. If compassion is really there in the room between the two of you, the client will feel it, and you can say pretty much anything to them because it is coming from a place of sensitivity and care.

I had a client who was ruining his life by gambling, and he knew it. It was very painful, but he had made progress. Then he gambled excessively on an online game. When he told me, I had an honestly disappointed reaction. He felt ashamed, but our relationship did not end. He knew I was still in it with him, and on some level, he knew that my reaction was honest. The work for us was for him to get in touch with his own disappointment as well and try to turn it into action. I was representing a voice that he needed to start embodying. I did not want him to become judgmental of himself, just to be more realistic. I tried to convey to this client that I understood his longing, how in that instant, he wanted to feel alive. I also wanted him to turn his shame into resolve. Maybe eventually, he could say for himself that he didn't want to gamble anymore.

This was painful for the client yet a relatively easy instance for the therapist of being compassionate and straightforward with a client. He knew that I was on his side while he struggled. Yet what if a client said something bigoted or racist in session? Social justice is a part of our work, and we need to react to offensive comments made by clients in session.

Perhaps in these situations, we might say something like, "I want to hear where that is coming from, but I can't sit here and say nothing." This might yield a confrontation in session, but if there is enough of an alliance established, it might withstand the requisite challenge to their thinking. If a client does not even realize that they are saying something biased, then you might need to bring it to their awareness in a timely and skillful way. What an opportunity it would be if the client is up for it! You could say, "It is hard for me to hear you say what you just said and I am concerned about where these beliefs stem from. I think I can help you, as there is important work that we could do together about what you just said. I am hoping we can work through what I am about to say here."

We do not necessarily want to *debate* the client about the content of their comment. We want to have a deeper *conversation* instead. It may feel a little heavy-handed to lecture them on what was offensive about their comment, yet it would likely be more therapeutic to speak your mind even if it means losing the case. Keeping the alliance by silently letting offensive comments be spoken would not be an honest foundation for therapy. We need to find a way to compassionately challenge bigotry right away in session. The trick is to try to get the alliance established quickly during the course of therapy. Remember, clients will have a distorted experience of you anyway. They do not take you in as a full person and might be surprised when you have your own reactions to what they share. Your work is to find the opportunity to bring what arises naturally within you during a session and turn it into therapeutic gold.

Chapter 8 Bibliography

1 Leonard, H. Kapelovitz, M.D. (1987). *To Love and to Work/A Demonstration and Discussion of Psychotherapy*. Northvale, NJ: Jason Aronson, p. 66.
2 Asch, S. (1958). *Journal of the American Psychoanalytic Association. II, 1954: Transference and Countertransference: A Historical Survey. Douglass W. Orr. Pp. 621-670, Psychoanalytic Quarterly, 27, 282*.
3 Sullivan, H.S. (1970). *The Psychiatric Interview*. Scranton, PA: Norton.

9

ADDRESSING DIMENSIONS OF CULTURE IN COUPLES COUNSELING

In this chapter, we address how we can work with dimensions of culture in couples counseling. For example, what do we do in premarital therapy when couples from different cultures navigate the challenges of creating their wedding? How do we address our own identity and cultural differences in the room with our clients? Can we increase our cultural competency and understand that a person's identity is how they define who they are? While there are many identities that can describe someone, there are some that are more salient than others. We take a look at the "Big 8" socially constructed identities: race, ethnicity, gender identity, (dis)ability, sexual orientation, religion/spirituality, nationality, and socioeconomic status.[1]

Dimensions of culture in couples counseling

If we are to be client-centered and tend carefully to presenting problems, then we need to be sure that we are constantly aware of dimensions of culture and identity in therapy. While clients might present with a

DOI: 10.4324/9781003283164-10

variety of issues that merge together, our ability to track how systems of oppression and aspects of race and ethnicity impact their experiences is critical in creating a safe space for change.

One thread that is present in all clinical cases is culture. Cultural competency is the degree to which we pay attention to and understand the impact of culture in our clinical work. Making explicit how a client's culture, race, ethnicity, and socioeconomic status might impact their experience of life is an important step. Putting words to our own identities is also paramount. If we address what is happening in the room and name how our own culture impacts how we work, we make room for differences to be honored.

For me, I am a white person who identifies as a straight, cisgender, heterosexual male. By naming that, I locate myself within a range of what Kimberlé Williams Crenshaw calls intersectional identities.[2] It also opens up room for the understanding that our identities shape how we understand and look at life's experiences. White men have been the cause of most of the world's problems throughout history. If a person of color comes to therapy with me, they very well may have negative associations with white men. I need to feel comfortable speaking to this dynamic with the client while constantly addressing within myself how my power and privilege show up in therapy. I also need to check with my client about how they identify and how their culture shapes their experiences and informs how they make sense of their life.

This goes double for couples counseling. With two people in the room, we need to find room to talk explicitly about their identities and how they impact their relationship. For instance, a couple navigating a ceremony such as a wedding, we could inquire about any traditions in their cultures. If you are working with an Armenian couple, then maybe you ask what an Armenian wedding looks like. You might know what Indian weddings look like or Jewish weddings, but assuming that you know the cultural aspects of an Armenian wedding without asking will cost you some opportunities to learn more about the couple. Instead, you might ask them directly to tell you what is involved in a wedding in their culture so that you would be more informed about the beliefs their culture has about relationships, weddings, and even love.

You cannot take culture out of it. Culture informs how a couple forms their identity. When an intercultural union is being formed, the couple must navigate the blending of their individual identities and form a unique, collaborative union. The couple's counselor might need to help the couple navigate the meaning of various practices. For instance, in one culture, removing your shoes when entering the house might have a specific meaning, while in another culture, that gesture does not matter. In some cultures where meaning is very much derived by gestures, also known as high context cultures, the rituals matter.[3] In a low context culture, meaning is derived more through words. It matters less what we do. It is more about the words we say. When an individual from a high context culture is in a relationship with an individual from a low context culture, they may need help understanding one another and how they make sense of love.

Actively addressing the unspeakable

We must attend to various identities such as culture, race, gender, and sexual orientation actively in the room. Naming the intersectional identities in the therapy room aligns with our overall task of naming and addressing various psychological phenomena in session. We need to get comfortable with addressing cultural differences in therapy as well. You may ask the clients, "What are your beliefs about relationships? Where do they come from? What did you see your parents do? Where are they from and what is their background?"

From the clients' answers, you might understand where your practice of couples counseling fits into their framework in terms of culture, race, and ethnicity. Included in this is how therapy itself is perceived where they are from and where their families are from. Is there shame about being in therapy that comes from cultural messages? Or is it widely accepted? Getting comfortable with making these questions explicit and talking about race helps honor the client's experience of life and challenges any assumptions that you might have about how they live and love.

Overtly expressing and challenging your assumptions and identifying how your experiences inform what you bring to your work is one way to make dimensions of identity speakable in the room. If you have a concern that talking about race or culture would illuminate something problematic and make therapy ineffective, then you need to work on leaning into your discomfort. Our implicit biases affect our work each session anyway. We all bring our biases informed by living in a white supremacist world. Instead of imposing our own worldview, it is incumbent on the culturally sensitive therapist to meet the couple where they are and learn about their beliefs. Saying where we are coming from – to be curious and open – makes for a more realistic and healthy ground for therapeutic work to occur. Additionally, there may be times when you share the same cultural background as a client, and you risk making too quick of an assumption that you are the same in every way. Sharing similar backgrounds can help build an alliance quickly, but we also need to be sure that we do not jump to any conclusions about a shared worldview.

Discussing dimensions of culture may bring it out of the subtext and to the surface, but we need to know how to continually address it as therapy unfolds. Developing your style of attending to race, ethnicity, gender identity, (dis)ability, sexual orientation, religion/spirituality, nationality, and socioeconomic status might help your clients get comfortable talking about it as well. You might have to make these definitions explicit, but you should also weave conversations about power and privilege into the flow of conversation. For example, say a client who immigrated to this country as a child is talking with you about the pressures at work. While their concerns are focused on their job, it can help to contextualize their experience by keeping their family of origin in mind and considering what work meant to them when they came to this country. This way, you are keeping in mind the presenting problem of work stress while also attending to the culturally informed messages about work that impact the client's experience, including what it means to have immigrated.

There may be times that you do not know enough about your client's culture and you might have questions. They may need to inform you about their experience, which could be healing for them in the sense that they experience your genuine curiosity. However, it also can cause exhaustion or fatigue for the client to have to teach you about their experience rather than your having a basic understanding to begin with. You should stay open and curious about how it is for the client to work with you and your potential blind spots, as it can be an important element in nurturing the therapeutic relationship.

For example, as a straight man, when I have worked with gay couples or queer individuals, there have been blind spots for me, and I have had to ask them to tell me more about what their experiences have been. While I was careful not to ask them to teach me, I also did not want to make assumptions. My hope was that they found my inquiries about their experiences in this world respectful rather than their feeling like they were working with a counselor who did not fully relate to or understand them. The hope was that in making our differences explicit it was building respect rather than causing a chasm. Relating across different dimensions of culture and navigating those differences is central to our work as clinicians.

We also need to deeply understand how power and privilege play out in the therapeutic relationship. Even if we have blind spots in this area, we must be willing to muddle through them and address the power that we hold in the role as *therapists*, as well as the power that we carry in our various identities. Rather than be silent in these conversations for fear that they will be uncomfortable or awkward, we need to lean into the discomfort and lay bare the impact of the power that we hold as the therapist. Not having the willingness to say anything can erode the therapeutic relationship. Even worse, it fortifies the power and privilege that we hold. Our fragility when it comes to these conversations can make us avoid addressing power dynamics because we are so afraid of being hurtful, yet avoiding conversations about differences reinforces the power dynamic and keeps it in place. Being able to tolerate when we get it wrong or when the client does not like what we have to say and not fall apart allows the client to safely talk to us about their experience with us and hopefully opens up a space for understanding and healing.

In couples counseling, this takes on even more importance. Addressing how power and privilege show up within the clients' relationship with one another and within the therapeutic relationship can help unlock painful feelings that may keep the couple stuck. Helping them talk with each other and with you about dimensions of identity can add a contextual lens to their presenting issues. They might find new insights and understanding about their situation when we talk about how race and culture might be affecting how they experience their relationship.

If the couple is from different backgrounds from each other, then you need to help them make sense of how those differences impact their patterns of relating. The messages about love and family that they bring to the relationship might need to be made explicit so that they can deepen their understanding and empathy for one another. Being a culturally sensitive and tuned-in therapist can help couples address their differences and bring to light how power dynamics and worldviews shape how they relate to one another. Maintaining a culturally informed lens with couples also allows space for those differences to be honored and for new patterns of relating to emerge.

Chapter 9 Bibliography

1   Johnson, A.G. (2006). Privilege, oppression, and difference. In *Privilege, Power, and Difference* (2nd ed., pp. 12–40). New York: McGraw-Hill.

2   Crenshaw, K. (1991). Mapping the margins: Intersectionality, identity politics, and violence against women of color. *Stanford Law Review, 43*(6), 1241–1299. doi:10.2307/1229039

3   Hall, E.T. (1959). *The Silent Language*. Garden City, New York: Doubleday & Company, Inc.

10

STARTING AND STOPPING WHO WE ARE: HOW TO BE YOURSELF AS A THERAPIST

In this chapter, we explore the difference between who we are in session and who we are out of the room. We also look in greater depth at what to do when we start and stop sessions. This transition is an important one, and we do our clients a great service when we better understand the impact of how we start and stop our work.

Self-disclosure

Each therapist has their preference and style when it comes to self-disclosure. The question in our field about self-disclosure is not purely about whether we should tell a client about what is going on in our lives. The question is more about how much of ourselves we should bring into the session. A deeper inquiry about self-disclosure centers around when we are being a therapist versus when we are being ourselves.

While many of us have a "therapist self" that comes through when we are in session, it can cause some dilemmas in terms of self-disclosure

DOI: 10.4324/9781003283164-11

when we keep our "real selves" out of the therapy process. If we blur that line so that there is not the "therapist self" and the "real self," then self-disclosure becomes less of a concern because we are always being ourselves when doing a therapy session. If you are going to work on being yourself in the room as a therapist, then you could also work on incorporating who you are as a therapist into your daily life. We just do not want a dramatic split between you as a therapist and you in your life. This can, of course, cause problems in your personal life because who in your life wants a therapist for a spouse, child, sibling, or friend?

If you are going to blur the line between self and therapist, then it has to go both ways. If I saw you at a concert, or dinner party, or on the playground somewhere, you should be similar to who you are in session. You might be highlighting different aspects of yourself, but those aspects should still be with you in therapy. All your aspects are in the therapy room and should be welcome because they might have something to offer to your client.

Conversely, if you were at a punk rock festival, the therapist in you would still be at the punk rock festival, but you would not be providing therapy there. Instead, you might be living with a certain lens of insight, depth, and feeling even while you are at the concert, maybe more so than the other punk rockers there. Similarly, your "punk rock self" could come with you to the therapy room. Typically we would say that our punk rocker has no place in therapy, but considering that we want to be ourselves wherever we go, perhaps a punk mindset of letting yourself be free could come in handy with some clients. If a client brings up something wild or edgy, the "punk rock" part of the therapist might be willing to go there, whereas another more conservative part of the therapist might have a more adverse reaction and would be less useful in that moment.

Bringing all of yourself into the room

The key to being yourself in the room and having self-disclosure come naturally is to be at ease with yourself. If the client experiences their therapist at ease, then they are more likely to engage fully in the process. If you bring self-compassion into the therapy process, then it will extend to your clients, and they will feel it. If you are hard on yourself and have a loud, critical inner voice, the client will feel this lack of ease and might feel less open to the therapy process.

A kind inner voice is the essence of self-care. If you are beating yourself up inside and then attempt to have a voice with your clients that is kind, then it will ring hollow because your loud inner critic may come through in how you speak to your client. How you speak to yourself will get transmitted to your client. We need to get the inner critic under wraps in order to have an effective and easy presence with our clients so that they feel our loving-kindness more than our criticism.

Your authentic self as the tool

The therapist is the instrument for the work, so the therapy itself will only go as far as you do. If you, as the instrument, are not well-tuned, then it does not matter how good your training is. The therapy will fall flat since you are out of tune. Focusing on being more authentic in your therapeutic relationships (in fact, all of your relationships) can be more impactful than added training that centers solely on interventions. If you focus too much on interventions and not enough on yourself as a therapist, you might miss the chance for more effective and sustainable work.

Therapists constantly edit their interventions because we measure what we say and how it will be received. We analyze how our interventions land, which then shapes our next intervention. It helps to pay attention to how that editing in the room differs from our self-editing outside of the room. When we are with family and friends socializing, we are also editing ourselves in terms of how we behave and what we say. Yet it is likely different than the editing we do as clinicians. We generally measure ourselves more self-consciously when we are socializing and more analytically when we are working.

As clinicians, we work to be more self-aware. We pay attention to what we say and do in the room, and this must also bleed into our personal lives because being a clinician will affect us and our relationships. We start to interact differently in our personal lives as we grow more self-aware of how we communicate and interact. The deeper conversations we are having with our clients will probably affect us and influence the conversations we have with others in our personal life. Our style of communicating may morph over the years both in and out of the room, and that is perfectly healthy.

The start of your sessions

If we are working toward being the same self before, during, and after sessions, then it might be useful for us to get clear about what happens within us when we start and stop sessions. Hopefully, we are still the same person when the session starts, but something usually shifts when we welcome the client into the session. There is a delineation between when the session starts and when it ends. What does that start and stop look like for you?

What happens before you open the door to start the session? Are you doing notes, writing emails, returning a phone call, caught up in your own stuff, running to the bathroom, eating a sandwich, and then it's suddenly the top of the hour, and it is time to start? Or does something subtle shift inside of you before you even open the door and greet the client? Delineating the mindset of being in session versus not being in session is an important shift. We may imagine softly asking ourselves if we are ready to tune everything out in our lives and be present with our client. We are being paid for our presence, so we should get ourselves prepared before we start the session. We need to be ready to be present when the session starts, and to do that, we might need to do something on the inside to delineate "on" and "off."

When people meditate, they sometimes ring a bell, light a candle, or burn incense to signal to themselves that they are meditating. The meditation ends, and they blow out the candle to signal that they are back to their normal waking consciousness. Even if the meditator is the same person when they are meditating and not meditating, they still benefit from delineating when they are "on" and "off." Could you, for your practice as a clinician, have something that signals to you that you are moving into the mindset of doing therapy? Even if it is the same you there in session, once it begins, you might be a little more consciously present than you were before. You may not need to light a candle or ring a bell, but you should have your own signal that you are ready to begin work.

I worry about myself when I bleed in and out of sessions. When I am in the middle of an email and it is time to start the session, but the email is not quite finished and I am not ready, it feels like I spill into the session in an unhealthy way. My body might be in the chair with the client, but my head is still over by my computer trying to finish that email. This sort of beginning feels blended and messy to me and does not seem like the best approach. Instead, I do better when I take a little time to get ready, to center myself, and then work on being with the client in a different way than I would if I were just hanging out in between sessions.

Ideally, the first thing I would say to the client each session is "So?" and the session starts from there. "So?" feels like a little invitation and suggests picking up where we left off last session. If I could even say less and just nod my head to the client, that would be even better, but usually, I will have to say something like "How are you?" to signal to them that we are starting. Yet I would love it if I were just able to say "So?" and the client would just take it from there. The "so" suggests to me that we are getting back in the river of therapy again.

To get to the place where you can jump back into the river with your client, you have to shut everything else off in your life. You have to tell everything else to stop because there is so much input we take on as competent people. We could be checking texts and emails, checking in at home, eating a quick snack and reading the news between sessions and then, without a break, open the door to greet our client. Many of us can easily do this and the client would be none the wiser. Yet I wonder what would happen to our sessions if we turned off all inputs for a few moments before the session starts, took a few deep breaths to center ourselves and then opened the door to our clients. Something different might happen when this extra space is created.

The session begins for the client when they leave their house to come to our office or when they leave their work to come to the session. For remote therapy, it starts when the client stops what they are doing and logs in for the call. They recognize that it is time to go to therapy and a shift happens within them. They might start wondering what they want to talk about or start to turn their attention to themselves in ways that they do not normally. To match this shift in the client, it would be nice if the therapist did their own recognition that the session is starting before they open the door. A shift in mindset makes a difference.

The end of your sessions

As mentioned, we want to do our best to be the same person in and out of session. Yet there is a marked starting and stopping of sessions. If done consciously, this border can help with the clinician's self-care. When the session starts, you shift your mindset and get to a place where you are quietly ready. Then there is the encounter with the client where we invite them into the process of therapy. Some work gets done and then it is time to wrap up and stop. Being conscious of how we stop the session and move out into the rest of our day where we are not working is very important.

We first want to be conscious of slowing down before stopping. A part of the work slows before you get into the final phase. You are not going for therapeutic gold with just 5 minutes left in the session. You stop uncovering or probing well before the session ends so that you do not open anything up that you cannot process before stopping. Being conscious that you are in the last 10–15 minutes of the session might help you pace the work so that it does not bleed over the time boundary. You would stop questioning and opening things up well before you move into the wrapping-up phase of the session.

Problems occur when the therapist feels insecure about not having done enough in the session. The insecure therapist realizes that there are 15 minutes left, but they worry that the client may not be satisfied. So out of the therapist's anxiety, they take it further than it needs to go. When the therapist should be decelerating, they gas it. They go more into the work rather than pulling out. Preparing to end the session, even if the work is not totally completed, can help you pump the breaks on your therapeutic session. Even if you did not get to where you needed to that session, sometimes less is more. Instead of taking the work right up to the time boundary, you may send a signal that it is time to start wrapping up. You slow down, pause, ask the client how the session has been, and start to wrap up. Then you signal that it is the end of the meeting.

Getting clear about how you mark that the session is stopping can give you a strong sense of how to manage this boundary.

What is your signal to end the session? You might say, "we have to stop," which externalizes the ending. The time is making us stop. If you say, "We should wrap up now," then it has more of a feel that the therapist is dictating the ending of the session. It may not be easy to know what to say when the session ends. Do you shout, "Time's up!"? Probably not. Usually, a better approach is when we send a non-verbal cue that the session is ending such as adjusting our posture, looking knowingly at the clock, or shifting our demeanor to show that we are saying goodbye. The client may feel that we are sending them a sign. Perhaps then maybe we say something like, "Okay, should we schedule our next meeting?" It might not feel as abrupt to talk about scheduling once you have changed your non-verbal posture. You could really say whatever you want to in order to end it, as long as a non-verbal cue has been sent and received.

Once it's clear that the time is up, it is time to cross the threshold from the therapy room into the rest of the world. The door opens and the client leaves. Or we log off of the remote therapy call. In crossing this threshold, do you open the door for the client when they leave? Or do they open their own door? Do you walk out with them to the waiting room, so they find their way out? Do you let them log off first, or do you leave the meeting and hang up?

In person, I tend to open the door but not go with them across the threshold into the waiting room. They leave on their own and I tend to leave the door open. If need be, I might close the door behind them, keeping me inside the room in case I am worried about their lingering on the boundary. I feel like I should see the client out and then let them find their way out of the office altogether.

Then a very sacred process begins when one session ends and another one may be starting again in 10 minutes. You have a little bit of time for yourself in which something important happens. You must find a way to end and cleanse the previous session, do a little something for yourself, and then get ready to start it all over again.

11

HOW DOES THAT MAKE YOU FEEL? PLEASE DON'T ASK THAT

In this chapter, we look at how we can help clients get more connected emotionally. Rather than asking, "How does that make you feel?" we can instead find creative, metaphorical, symbolic, and transactional ways to help a client map out their internal world and reclaim what might have been lost when they previously disconnected from their emotional self. We also meander into the meaty question of whether the mind is in the body or the body in the mind, along with a few other metaphysical conundrums.

Getting emotionally connected

If there is one thing we know about working closely with people, it is that if you go right at their issues, you are going to meet their defenses. Being direct or asking the questions, "How does that make you feel?" and "What are you feeling?" usually cause clients to shut down or just report some thoughts about their feelings rather than actually feel the

DOI: 10.4324/9781003283164-12

feeling. Occasionally, if I notice emotions in the room, or if the patient is about to cry, I might just ask, "What is happening right now?" That usually elicits some emotion in those moments. Yet unless I see the welling up of feelings, I do not go charging into the client's emotional world because I do not want to meet their resistance and defensiveness directly.

Usually, there is a sort of circuitous approach I take, where I try to talk tangentially around a topic so that it might elicit some of the feelings. Emotions are invisible, and for most people, their inner worlds are not mapped out very well. Our job is to make the invisible visible. We, as humans, do not see emotions, so our work is to help the client look inside themselves into a world that is invisible.

How do we make the invisible visible when it comes to emotions? One way is by doing symbolic and transactional work in session. Beyond just naming feelings, we want the client to interact with their inner self in new ways. Since the inner world is invisible, we usually need to utilize abstract approaches. Using a person's imagination allows the invisible to become a bit more visible via their mind's eye. For many, their inner emotional lives are a big hairball – just a whole bunch of twisted up feelings. When we simply talk about emotions, we pull a thread of that hairball which we really do not know what it is connected to. Helping a client see the hairball in its entirety may be a safer and more holistic approach.

Instead of blithely asking, "How does that make you feel?" try instead to find a creative way to make a discussion of emotions symbolic, transactional, or interactive. Perhaps you might ask the client about their head versus their heart as a way of deepening the discussion. Of course, when you ask about the head or the heart, you are referring to an archetypal aspect of the person's being, not their cranium or the organ in their chest. We might ask a client, "You are talking a lot about what you think about this relationship, but what is going on in your heart?" This is a different way of asking how they feel, and it gives the person a better sense of where to start exploring their emotions.

Essentially, when it comes to emotions, we want to craft a language or road map for the client's inner life. You co-create a language with them. The words that you find are used to help the client reflect on what is happening on the inside. Having words to map out what is going on in one's inner world allows us to become more connected with those around us. Yet without the words, it can be much more challenging to share our inner self with others and to understand what is happening inside of them.

The missing affect

Sometimes your role as a clinician is to add the missing affect that the client is not feeling. Helping to heighten and name emotional experiences can go a long way toward cultivating depth. There is usually treasure in our emotional selves. Yet if somebody has spent decades defending themselves against their emotions, they are not going to start emoting within a couple of sessions with you. It might even take them many months before they start feeling their feelings. If you are dealing with decades of defenses that have worked to keep your client from accessing emotions, then you have your work cut out for you. Just because you ask them what they are feeling does not mean that the client is instantly going to be able to express it.

We should operate from a supposition that there is treasure in our emotions; that being in touch emotionally helps us reclaim lost power, lost wisdom, lost ability, and a lost sense of connection with ourselves in the world. If we connect to our emotional self, we open up a host of possibilities for living a more fulfilling life. It is important and brave work, almost like an archeologist of the inner planes of existence, helping the person go inside and get more connected.

If helping a client get in touch emotionally is challenging, then you might want to focus on meaning-making. This can be a step on the way toward being in touch emotionally. You frame the journey to emotion by helping the client make sense of their emotional life. You might talk about feeling the feelings before you even help the client actually *feel* their feelings. Preparing to feel is a good step. Perhaps the client might not access their emotions in that session, but we could help them get ready to become more in touch with feelings.

For a client who is more in their head, you likely will need to discuss with them symbolically what it would be like for them to go into their heart. It is not going to feel good to go into the heart, but we may just take little steps as we get more connected to our feelings. We touch into them and then move out. The key here is to talk about what we will eventually do in the future so that the client gets prepared to start feeling. This is all symbolic talk, not an actual heightening of emotions. It is our use of metaphor that can help with mapping out the client's inner life. A journey toward feelings takes patience and creativity, but it is well worth it.

Externalizing archetypes

Using metaphors to help people understand their feelings can be an efficient way of deepening the therapeutic process. When you talk with a client about their inner child, their shadow, or perhaps their angry self, you are talking about archetypal aspects of the person. You are naming a collection of thoughts and feelings that lie within them. Obviously, we are not going to cut the client open and see an inner child pop out. The archetypal aspects are a collection of thoughts, feelings, reactions, and beliefs about ourselves, as well as how we interpret the world.

We can push these inner processes out and form them into an entity of sorts so that we might relate to it. Whatever comes up with a client, we can create a language around it (your inner bully, your angry guy, your teenage self) so that the client might see themselves differently. The way you use language helps shape the experience of therapy for the client. You can say something that helps the client see within more effectively.

For instance, you could say, "You know, every time you talk about your family another aspect of you emerges. This aspect feels slippery and elusive. We were just talking about your family and now we are talking about politics instead. Have you noticed that you have this slippery aspect of yourself?"

Saying something like this unveils the client's avoidance, yet it can also help them feel your compassion. If you ask about this slippery aspect of them rather than directly challenging the client's avoidant behavior, then they may be more likely to open up. They may be more willing to play with you in the realm of inner emotions.

Maybe the client would respond, "Yeah, I have always done that. In high school they called me Sneaky Sam because I would always sneak out of the conversation." You then, of course, might ask, "What are we going to do with this Sneaky Sam guy? He shows up here in our work, but I bet he shows up in all of your relationships." Now, we are off to the races because we just had an opening to create a different way of relating with the client's inner sense of self.

When a client has a lot of unaddressed emotion running their life, we want to get it out from under the surface so that it can be processed. In most people's subconscious, they hold a collection of mixed-up feelings that they don't understand. Picking out one aspect of the emotional self and naming it can change the relationship the client has with their inner life. The emotional work starts when the client begins to relate to, for example, their slippery self. They might start to understand where Sneaky Sam was born, what its function is, and where it came from. The client might even say thank you to Sneaky Sam for getting them out of all sorts of uncomfortable situations. It could be your job as the compassionately challenging therapist to change what the dialogue is between the client and their emotional archetypal self.

The model of going deeper

Taking on the various aspects of the inner self is not something that most people choose to do willingly. They end up having to look within because aspects of their life are not working. They may have tried to change their behavior or their thinking but still have not seen desired results. Therapy is a kind of a failure-driven model. If we could just create behavioral change and see results, we would stop there. We would have no reason to do more work. However, if changing our behavior does not fix the problem, then therapy needs to shift toward working on changing cognition. Hopefully, we will see alleviation from presenting symptoms once the cognition changes. If changing the way we think fixes the problem, then we do not need to look inside any further. Yet if we are still stuck, then we may need to go deeper into emotions. If that fails, then we have to keep going deeper. Mapping this process out for people can help them understand why we are even asking about feelings. In therapy, we need to talk about why we are even going to go toward emotions before we just start going there. We need to set up a rationale for why we need to start looking within.

The reason we need to create this rationale is that most people are what we could call head-blind. They do not have their inner lives mapped out. As clinicians, we need to consider that most of us are half asleep and that our awareness has not been attuned to look inside ourselves. We learn from an early age to tune out what is happening within. Painful experiences cause us to dial down our awareness of what is going on within us. We go on autopilot in order to cope.

People come to therapy because eventually, the pain they have buried comes to the surface. If they are in enough pain, they might be willing to look within and start doing something differently. They need to learn what it means to go within. When we talk about going within, we don't just mean within the body. Although feelings are in the body, we are talking about an aspect of the mind that tends to the inner self rather than the outer world.

If we are helping clients look inside themselves and better understand their internal world, including their feelings, then we should be clear about what we are referring to. What do we mean when we ask someone to look inside themselves? If people are head-blind, how are we supposed to help them to become more aware? We can consider that "inside" versus "outside" are different dimensions. They are different levels of what is happening in life. If we can get people to start to wake up to the life happening inside of them, rather than thinking that all of life is outside of them, then it can give the client additional freedom and understanding of themselves. Most of us are trained to go out and try to find connection outside of ourselves. Yet it helps to train ourselves to feel connected on the inside so that we are able to help others do the same.

Clients will give you little clues along the way that are doorways into emotional work that can be done. Asking them what they feel is a heady way to go there and will likely be met with resistance. Instead, we want to look for metaphors and help the client relate differently to their inner world. We can create a story and landscape with the client and help them map out their lives. I encourage you to try to go there with clients when the opening presents itself.

12

NAMING YOUR SHADOW AND GRAPPLING WITH THE UNKNOWN

This chapter looks at how we deal with difficult presenting issues such as grief and loss, as well as how we sit with existential mysteries and the unknown with our clients. Perhaps one answer is to take on our own understanding of why bad things happen to good people and get a sense of why we feel we must provide answers for our clients. Maybe one more lasting solution is to go deeper into ourselves and do our own shadow work so that we can sit more comfortably with life's mysteries. We end up seeing in a new way that we can only take our clients as far as we are willing to go.

Addressing the deeper questions

As clinicians, we hear horrible stories from our clients. Stories of being abused or deeply neglected as children, or sudden traumatic events occurring in their adult lives. It is challenging to sit with clients who have experienced horrific events and figure out what you are going to say

DOI: 10.4324/9781003283164-13

that might be helpful. The underlying question the client is asking is, *why did this horrible thing happen to me?* When a trauma befalls a client, there is no easy substantive answer for "Why me?" We might wonder why suffering happens or why bad things occur, yet it can be difficult to know how to actually help the client when they have faced something overwhelming.

You would be shortsighted as a clinician if you did not take on a philosophical inquiry into why suffering happens to people in the first place. We are not philosophers or religious scholars, but as clinicians, we need to clarify our thinking about life's struggles. Just as we need to be steeped in current events and culture, we also need to be doing our own workaround wrestling with life's great mysteries. It can come out of nowhere when a client brings up an existential question. A client that you have been working with for a while might disclose past traumas that you were not expecting. You need to be ready to go to deeper existential places with your clients at a moment's notice.

Some of the traumatic events that happen to us have an existential element to them. Questions about why bad things happen in life in the first place and wondering if the world is a bad place are normal responses to trauma. Scholars, philosophers, mystics, and religious leaders have been taking on these inquiries for thousands of years, generation after generation, and it is still a mystery. We do not have answers to these weighty questions, yet as therapists, we are called to wrestle with these topics in session with our clients. If the scholars and mystics could not figure it out, then why do we think we would all of a sudden have answers?

Our clients may look to us for answers, yet rather than try to come up with them, we ought to focus instead on knowing what our relationship is to those mysterious questions themselves. If we do not know what our stance is, nor what our relationship is to existential realities, we are likely going to hit uncomfortable edges where we avoid going there with clients. Our goal is to try to safely go to scary emotional places with clients, even if we still do not have an answer. We may find ways to explore or map out life's mysteries. We can learn how to openly inquire about why bad things happen to good people, or why people suffer, or why there is loss, and even what happens when we die. Being able to have those conversations helps the therapeutic process. We should consider that underneath every single session is a question about life and death.

We care about the content that clients bring to session, yet we know that beneath what they are talking about are deeper unknowns.

When you have no answers

Since we do not have answers to the deeper unknowns, we can practice not knowing. My best two months of therapy, measured by experiences in the room, symptom relief and responses from clients, were when I was coming off of a horrible breakup. I was heartbroken and really not okay for two months. Yet it was the best two months for me as a therapist because I had no answers for clients. I had no capacity to solve everyday problems and find solutions. Instead, I sunk down into not knowing and was able to be present in session in much more impactful ways.

Where I normally might have wanted to take a solution-focused, problem solving, answer giving, strategizing approach to session, I was left to take a less heady and more heartfelt approach in session when life's events were too overwhelming. In my two months post-breakup, I could not provide any useful solutions or recommendations. When people brought up their struggles, I was more open-hearted (brokenhearted, actually) and in the muck with them. I was likely much more compassionate during that time than I might have been otherwise because I had no answers to give. All I could do was be there with the clients and sit there. Doing so allowed for other things to occur in the room.

Without having to be overwhelmed or traumatized by life, you might find yourself being more effective if you made some space for not having the answers to your client's questions. In this line of work, it is your ability to be in the unknown that makes you more competent. You do better when you can sit with the mystery and not try to solve your clients. Perhaps instead, you could find faith in the clients' ability to find solutions themselves. What if you trusted your clients' wisdom even when they are going through something difficult? Might that make your job just a bit easier?

What I often hear from clients who have had really poor experiences with previous therapists is that they experience their past therapist not saying very much of value. For instance, a client disclosed a real struggle, and the therapist did not know what to say. The client gave up on the therapist or felt outraged that the therapist provided some simple plati-tude in response. When I hear this sort of story from clients, I know it is not the previous therapist's fault that they did not know what to say. It can be difficult to find the words in the face of our clients' suffering. It is usually when their level of pain triggers our own pain that we lose the capacity to know what to say. In these moments, the client desperately wants to feel our compassion. Our work is to find ways of conveying that compassion, if even with a few heartfelt words.

Transforming your shadow

To process your own pain, so you are more comfortable sitting with your clients' pain, it means looking at the aspects of yourself that are often hidden. Uncovering and healing your own hurts can be a painful process, but it helps your clients. It is more beneficial for the client if their therapist is in the process of figuring out their own struggles. If the client were doing therapy with a perfect machine, then their therapeutic material would not be met with the needed humanity that it takes to heal their wounds. Being in a relationship with another human being who is imperfect and figuring it out is more healing than being with some-one who has it all together. It actually makes the therapy better when you allow yourself to be in the process of transformation and growth. Indeed, if a client were to go to a machine and tell the machine what was going on in their life, the machine might spit out the right answer, but it would not be nearly as helpful as sitting with another person who is on the same journey of life. The relationship with another human being who can honestly relate to life's struggles ends up having a more far-reaching impact than a solution.

You can only take your client as far as you are willing to go. The essence of "self of the therapist" work is that when we are working on ourselves, we become the instrument that carries the therapeutic infor-mation into the room and into the client's life. You could do all the required reading in graduate school and be up to speed on all the current research, but if you are not doing developmental work on yourself, then it would not matter because the art of therapy demands refining yourself as the instrument of the work.

Where this work really has an impact on your client is when you can do your own shadow work. Shadow work is scary and takes courage, but it also provides a bedrock of healing for your clients. If you can train yourself to be like a first responder who runs *toward* the danger rather than flees from it, then you might learn to be more comfortable with what is scary in life. When you incorporate aspects of your identity that often do not fit with being a therapist, then you know you are deepening your capacity to connect with aspects of humanity that are not always very lovely.

The key is to acknowledge where you are rigid about your self-concept and expand it to include all aspects of what it means to be human. If you consider yourself generous and compassionate, then you might need to note that you also have the capacity to be cruel and withholding. If you encounter a couple and one of the partners is cruel and withholding, then you will be able to work with them more effectively if you have worked with aspects of yourself that are cruel and withholding. For if you did not do that work, you might end up being more judgmental of the other person who shows up as cruel and withholding. You would likely say something that is not as compassionate as it could be and cause a rift in the therapeutic relationship.

We need modalities of practice that help us go into our shadow because most forms of healing conspire to take us out of it. We need mentors and supervisors who care enough about our development that they can point out what we are avoiding in ourselves and in our work. Therapeutic practices that help us access the stuck and twisted places with us and that help us get unstuck can be more successful than others when it comes to shadow work. We would call this work a modern-day alchemy, transforming psychological lead into gold. Taking your shadow, becoming more aware of it, confronting it with compassion, and transforming it so that it is incorporated into who you are allows for more effective and productive therapy.

The transmutation of your shadow might be the best thing that you can do for your clients, especially in helping them through tough emotional times. We can certainly be with them as a witness and companion through their journey. But to be a true instrument of healing and transformation, we need to do the work to touch the depths of ourselves.

13

PUTTING THOUGHTS INTO WORDS: HOW FINDING YOUR VOICE HELPS WITH CLINICAL CONFIDENCE

This chapter focuses on finding your voice which goes way beyond what you say in session and extends deeper into clarifying how you think. Grounding yourself in your theory of change can help with clinical confidence and give you a clearer sense of what to do with the "I don't know what to do" feeling.

What to do when you don't know what to say

I often hear from therapists both new and experienced that they feel like they do not know what they are doing. It can be very overwhelming to be in this position, not feeling equipped or properly trained to handle a presenting problem or clinical situation. When you encounter something in therapy that you have never faced before, you can feel like a deer in headlights. This paralysis is doubly felt when your client is looking to you for help right then.

DOI: 10.4324/9781003283164-14

When clients ask you either directly or indirectly how to handle various situations in their lives, what do you do in those moments that actually adds value? Therapy gets a bad rap, deservedly so when the therapist says something devoid of substance in response to the client's plea for help. The therapist might ask the client what they have previously tried, or they explore what gets in the way of the client finding answers, but the client wants something substantive when they ask for help. They do not want a redirect.

If the client asks you what to do about a situation that you have never dealt with before, personally or professionally, it is difficult to know what to say other than redirecting them back to their own ideas about what to do. For instance, if a client says that their ex-spouse is taking them back to court because of financial disagreements, they want your help with knowing what to do. Unless you have been in this situation or have particular training and experience with divorced couples and financial arrangements, you might not be able to relate to and know what to say. You could counsel them to slow down and find ways of deescalating. Yet the client is looking for clarity about what to do about their financial situation. Not giving them what they are looking for likely leaves them feeling disappointed and perhaps questioning therapy overall.

What do you do if you are faced with the feeling of not being sure what to say in session or how to intervene? One thing you can do is to say to the client something like, "You strike me as a very smart person. If this were easy for you to solve then you would have figured this out already. Of course you want to come here and get an answer. If it were that easy to give you an answer, you would have found it through your own resources. This situation is much messier. Therapy is a process by which we are going to find an answer together."

The key here is to not just say something just for the sake of it. You don't want to fill the room with empty words just because the client expects you to have answers to their questions. You want to try to be on your word, where there is meaning to what you say. You want there to be a sense that you are present and aware of what you are saying, as opposed to being somewhere else when you speak. You may find yourself scrambling to talk because the client is expecting you to respond with something to say. You might even watch yourself talk just to be speaking. Yet try to resist the pull to say something that is just words in order to fill the void.

Before you know what to say to your client, you can ask them a delaying question in order to gather more information. You could find something in the moment that helps the client feel oriented, held, and met while you organize your thinking. You could ask them for more details while you formulate your hypothesis and plan out what you are going to say next. One aspect of being an effective therapist is having a lightning quick mind. You have to be either one step ahead of your client, or you have to be ready to quickly conceive of something to say that has substance. I do not know how you train your mind to necessarily work more quickly. Your words might go more slowly when you do not know what to say, but your mind has to quickly filter through a lot of data and figure out what you want to say that is going to help the work move forward.

When you do not know what to say, and when your insecurity starts to tell you, "I do not know what I am doing. I do not know how to treat this person. I do not know how to help cure them. I have not seen this before. I do not know what to do," then it helps to return to what your theory of change is. If you are not sure how to solve the presenting problem or what to say to help, then you could at least start by knowing your theory of change. Perhaps you believe that change happens in relationships. If that is the case, then when you do not know what to say about a particular presenting problem, you might say something to the client that conveys that you are it with them. You could express your care for them. If you believe that change happens through learning new information, then perhaps in a moment of uncertainty, you might say to your client, "I do not know the answer, but let me do some research and consult with a colleague." If your theory of change says that healing happens when someone's problems are witnessed by another person, then you might say something like, "Let me share my thoughts about what I am noticing about your situation."

In those moments, it can be very useful to slow down to get your thoughts together. The quicker your mind works, the easier it will be, but it's okay if the client sees you slowing down and thinking. Over time you might find clear ways of knowing what to say that will move the clinical work forward.

What are you thinking?

It can be especially challenging to know what to say when a client asks you what they should do. They want advice and ask something like, "What do you think I should do in this situation?" In those moments, the client is actually asking two separate things: "What do you think?" and "What should I do?" You might not have a clue.

When a client asks what you think, you could strongly consider telling them. However, when they ask what they should do, start with telling them what you are thinking because you might not really know what they "should" do. For instance, you might reply with something like, "Here is what I am hearing. I hear that you are very anxious. I know it is difficult when you are not sleeping. I see this all the time with my clients. I know it can be very overwhelming."

Whatever it is you are thinking, your task is to try to find a useful way to share it. If it is a negative thought you are having, then you want to figure out how to share that thinking in a way that is not raw, but that forms itself into an intervention. For example, if you think to yourself, "This guy is so helpless, always such a victim," you rephrase it as something more compassionate about how you can appreciate struggling and feeling helpless.

If a client asks for your advice about what to do, just take a second and tell them what you are hearing first. There is no way you are going to gather all the experience and data and information of what goes on for people in their lives to have a full set of answers about how to advise them on what they should do. You are not going to have every single human problem figured out. That is not the goal. Yes, you might gain specialties and categories of knowledge over the course of your career. You might have even seen a theme before with previous clients and have a sense of what tends to help them. But you are not trying to answer clients' questions for them, nor tell them what to do to solve their problems.

Instead, if you are going to practice in a relational way, in a client-centered way, you must find ways to share your honest thoughts about the situations in clients' lives to get them on the path toward health and wellness. The goal is to resource your client, to help them gain a stronger sense of self, and to help them get out of a reactive emotional place in order to start thinking clearly again. You just need to be able to do that for yourself first.

Provide substance, not problem-solving

Rather than fixing the client, we want to help them become self-actualized – more effective, more in touch with their emotions, more skillful, more aware. Oftentimes, it does not really matter what the presenting problem is. The goal is to have the person develop in the face of their problem. You are not seeing the forest or the trees when you just see the presenting problem and a treatment plan. When you get into that sort of mindset, then the presenting problems become like a game of whack-a-mole. A problem pops up, and you jump to try to solve it. Your clients will come in with a new problem the following session and forget about the last problem they were talking about last week. Your goal is to take whatever life is sending their way and figure out what growth is available for them in it.

A breakup is a great example of this. When the client comes in and is going through a horrible, messy breakup, they are very focused on the problem. Their heart has been broken and torn out. They might read you text message exchanges between them and their ex. They might have it all printed out for you to read, or they will hand you their phone. They want you to know all the gory details of the breakup so you might help fix the situation. In those moments, I will dive in and join them. "Oh my goodness, let me look at these messages!"

I am in all the details with them, but I do not really have a horse in that race. I am not focused on getting them back together with their ex or not. Instead, I am taking advantage of the opportunity for personal growth and development that might become available. A breakup is painful, yet it is often a great occasion for learning about ourselves. We get to see more clearly how we function in terms of loss, love, and attachment. We see more clearly the patterns that we replay in a relationship that we need to change.

As a therapist, you do not have to worry as much about the content of the presenting problem. Just remember that the substantive part of the work is the personal growth. Keep an eye on the growth potential for clients. Maybe they need to learn to be more brave. Maybe they need to learn to face their past or to be more compassionate or not beat themselves up too much. Keep an eye on personal growth. It will allow you to cut through to what the real therapeutic question is.

14

THE UNTAUGHT LESSONS OF PROFESSIONAL IDENTITY

This chapter explores professional identity and how we might find a way of conveying what we do in session to those outside the room. Graduate school focuses on learning the theory and practice of counseling and often does not have ample time to teach new clinicians about professional identity. As a result, we have to learn how to cultivate a professional presence that communicates to others what we are like in session. We can take our professional identities out into marketing and networking situations to generate more referrals. We can also be ambassadors for the profession conveying to others that going to therapy is a worthwhile pursuit.

Learning the lessons not taught in graduate school

It takes time and practice to learn the craft of therapy. Any person-centered or relational model of therapy takes years to develop. Instead of a manualized approach, learning the art of therapy requires practice and many hours of clinical work. Because of this, when graduate students ask

DOI: 10.4324/9781003283164-15

their supervisors or professors how to handle certain clinical situations, the answer from those supervisors almost always is, "It depends."

It depends on the various factors of the case. There is no manualized answer. If a student asks if they should meet with a client twice a week because the client requests it, then the supervisor's response is usually, "It depends." It depends on the presenting problem, how the weekly sessions are already being used, and if twice a week therapy is clinically indicated. There is no pat answer or blanket statement in response to this sort of question. Similarly, if a student therapist asks if they should bring their client's spouse into session to talk about their primary client's depression, then the answer also is, "It depends." It depends because there are so many variables to consider and bringing the spouse in would depend on the specifics of this case.

Because of this variability, graduate school is primarily focused on the theory and practice of counseling and on case consultation. Time and resources go into training the student how to do the basics, how to manage cases and to start to think about clients and trust their own decision making. There is little to no time to discuss professional identity or how the therapist plans to go out in the world after graduation and market their skills. A discussion of professional identity would be premature in graduate school, and most new therapists have very little sense of how they want to present themselves to prospective clients and places of employment once they graduate.

Professional identity

As we move into the field, we need to learn what professional identity is. Simply put, professional identity is how we convey to the outside world what we do in session. Other than our clients and perhaps our supervisors, nobody else knows what we are really like in session. It is a private process, and what we say and do is usually only experienced directly by our clients. In order to convey to others what we are like as a therapist, we need a persona, or professional identity, that transmits what we are all about. To let potential clients and referring therapists know what it is like to work with us, we have to develop a way of carrying ourselves and communicating our style of practice.

Graduate school does not have the time to teach us how to write a website bio or Psychology Today profile. Seldom do we learn in school how to network or how to give an elevator pitch about the way we practice. We might not even know our area of focus or the presenting problems and populations that we want to specialize in at first. As a result, most new therapists market themselves as generalists and find it hard to differentiate their practices from others. Why would a referring therapist refer to a new clinician rather than someone seasoned that they already knew? Developing a professional identity can help in this situation and can let others know what one's practice is really about.

Networking and marketing

At networking events, I have talked with countless therapists who have aimed to describe their practice and convey who they are as practitioners. They are often looking to cultivate referral sources and find new clients for their practices. One quick way for them to communicate the sort of clients that they want sent their way is to describe the presenting problems and populations they specialize in. They might talk about working with teens, eating disorders, or couples. They might have a focus on the LGBTQ or queer community or with a geriatric population. Whatever they say, it gets me thinking about the types of clients that I might send their way and how I can keep them in mind for future referrals.

Too many therapists, however, when asked to describe their practice, will give vague, general descriptions that make it difficult for others to think of them for referrals. These therapists will typically describe their practice as one that focuses on anxiety and depression, and that they work with adults and kids, and that they can work with couples … and men … and women … and so on. The point here is that they say that they can do everything, which very well be true, but it ends up giving no clear sense of what they are really like as clinicians. Of course, most of us can work with all sorts of clients and all types of presenting problems. Yet it is important that we learn to quickly convey the core of what we do so that we can transmit to others what it would be like to work with us in session.

At a networking event, it helps if you can hone in on the specifics of what you do and how you practice. What can set you apart and help define your practice is, expressing a unique key element of who you are as a clinician. If you are good at working with trauma cases, then it is useful to let others know about that area of focus. If you are trained to work with couples and families, then craft a brief pitch about how that training has helped you manage the challenge of working with more than one person in the room. This will go a long way toward communicating to others what you are about.

My pitch

When I was starting out, I would tell people that I work with men. My first client was a young man in the police academy, and right from there, I kept receiving referrals for individual male clients. I quickly found a way to create a connection with these clients, make the process of therapy comfortable for them, shoot the breeze a bit, and then take the conversation to more therapeutic levels. While I certainly felt comfortable working with women (and had many female clients, couples, and families already on my caseload), at networking events, the pitch I would give about my practice was that I work with dudes.

"Send me your dudes," I would say in those early networking events. "Think of me for your male clients. Send me your blue collar guys, your cops, construction workers, and police officers. I work with all sorts of male clients who might not be comfortable with the process of therapy. Send me your white collar guys too. Lawyers, executives, and guys stuck in their heads are my specialty. Please think of me for those cases."

People would laugh at first when I would talk about working with "dudes," but then they would get what I was trying to convey when I went on to talk more about working with men. I would discuss the particular challenges of getting through to men who are socialized to avoid putting their thoughts and feelings into words. Many of the clinicians at those networking events would reach out to me with referrals for not just individual male clients but also for couples where a male client was resistant. The key here was for me to be able to define a small niche and convey that niche effectively to others.

Conveying who you are

Beyond transmitting what you do in session, you also need to be able to convey who you are as a person. It does not matter how clearly you express your clinical interest and your preferred presenting problems and populations, if who you are as a clinician, and as a person does not come through in your professional identity, then your practice may remain a mystery to others and risks becoming detached from the outside world. While what we do in session is confidential, we need a bridge to the outside world to let others know about the work we are doing in private. Who you are as a person is that bridge. If you can bring a sense of yourself as a therapist to your interactions with others outside of session, then they can feel what it would be like to work with you.

For instance, if you are a quick-thinking clinician, able to identify problems and offer plausible solutions in session, then perhaps you can bring those qualities to your interactions with others in the outside world. Not just at a networking event but even at a cocktail party, you might find ways of transmitting this quick-thinking part of you. Not that you will be solving other people's problems at the cocktail party or giving free therapy over a glass of merlot. Instead, you might just share a bit of how you think about general world events or situations occurring in vivo at the cocktail party. However you do it, the practice of everyday professional identity is to naturally transmit who you are both in and out of session so that others experience what a therapist is like as a person. Many people have misconceptions about counseling and mental health practitioners. Being able to have a human experience with you can give them new data about what counseling can be like.

I try to keep this process in mind when socializing. I think that I am a warm, compassionate, and empowering therapist in session. I hope that I also convey those qualities in my everyday interactions. A bit of who I am as a therapist should come through in my day-to-day life, just as who I am as a person should show up in session. In this sense, putting my professional identity into action would mean taking my therapist self and projecting it out into the world in appropriate and useful ways. This does not mean that I would try to solve people's problems on the bus or ask someone about their childhood at a dinner party. Instead, the intention would be to have my conversations out of session contain some of the connectedness and depth of a therapy session. This way, when others experience me, they might have a positive experience about talking with another person who makes their living as a therapist.

Ambassadorship

I have heard of therapists generating referrals wherever they go. They enter into conversations with people in all sorts of situations, and the topic of being a therapist comes up. If done naturally, not from a sales pitch perspective, any conversation can lead to a referral. Checking out at the register of a retail store, in an elevator, at a wedding, traveling on an airplane ... all of these types of interactions can be a chance for us to subtly convey what the therapeutic process is all about.

More than just selling ourselves, we are also ambassadors for the profession. We convey to others not just what we are like in session but also what a therapist is like in general. Hopefully, we are grounded and human and relate a sense of lived wisdom that causes others to consider that therapy could be good for them. Our goal is to be relatable enough that people see therapy as an approachable process that can add value to their lives. An encounter with us can open the door to their therapeutic journey.

When I tell people that I meet for the first time that I am a therapist, the responses range. Some people respond with a joke, asking if I can read their minds or if I want to know what they are feeling. Others tend to shut down, and I can tell that they are uncomfortable talking with me. Another group of people respond with curiosity and might even start telling me about their own experience with therapy. Pretty quickly, I can tell what type of interaction it will be by the person's first response when the topic of what I do for a living comes up. Some people respect the profession and see it as a noble undertaking. Others are skeptical and approach the conversation with caution. Regardless of the response, I try to focus on ambassadorship, and while not doing any therapeutic work outside of session, I try to see if I can open the door a bit so that the other person can take a step closer to their own therapeutic process.

One way that we can make a difference in this world is by helping the people in it grow and change. If we touch one life in session, then it very well might ripple out into the rest of the world. Let us consider that even out of session, being a therapist in the world can make a difference. I try to keep in mind that if a person that I meet went to therapy and worked on themselves that they would likely become a little more connected with themselves. Their family might become a little more connected as well. Eventually, the connection might spread to their community, and the impact can ripple out from there.

15

A WORD OF ADVICE: DON'T GIVE ADVICE

In this chapter, we explore more fully what to do when clients ask for advice. We do not want to fall into the trap of trying to give advice and solve their problems, yet we also do not want to totally abandon them and leave them to fend for themselves. This chapter looks at potential situations when advice should be given and examples of when it should not. We also look more closely at what change looks like for our clients and how we conduct ourselves when they are resistant to change.

What to do when a client asks for advice

Building on our last chapter, when we explored what to do when we are unsure of what to say, we should be even more fully prepared when clients ask us for advice. What do you do when a client comes in and says, "I could use advice about to what to do in this situation?" Do you try to solve their problem for them? Do you tell them that you cannot

DOI: 10.4324/9781003283164-16

give them advice? These are tough situations when a client has a concrete question that needs answering or when they genuinely seek guidance. It is different from when they say that they are feeling stuck. Oftentimes clients will ask our opinion, and we can turn it back to them to help them find answers. For instance, as we explored a bit last chapter, if a client is going through a breakup and comes in asking for *support*, it is perhaps easier to know what to do as a clinician. You can help them find healthy ways to stay connected to life. Yet when they ask for advice about how to *handle* the breakup, we can feel paralyzed, not knowing exactly what to say.

Being asked for advice tugs on the part of us that wants to dispense our opinion. It can be hard to resist. You might even feel like you could guide them to make a good decision and have some sound advice that might make a difference. It helps to keep in mind that what makes us different as mental health practitioners is that our focus is to help others find their own answers rather than give them ours. The goal is to facilitate the emergence of solutions from their own innate wisdom rather than foster a dependency on others for direction in life. This is different from writing into an advice column where the columnist is going to give a direct solution to the problem.

The problem for clinicians is when a client is in distress and wants advice in the moment to help relieve their pain. They do not want to tolerate the process of the therapist eliciting information from them and getting them to find their own way. That is a slower process and may not feel as good for them in the moment as being guided by the advice of a professional. It can be seductive to tell the client what to do when they are in distress in order to help them feel more stable. Yet if you give advice and it is the wrong advice (in the sense that they do not see the results they are looking for or it causes them more pain), you set yourself up for hurting the therapeutic alliance. You might cause more damage because you may not have the full picture.

I typically try to stay out of the advice-giving business, but I can relate to wanting advice from somebody who might have more wisdom than me or who can see more clearly than I do. It fits into an age-old tradition of going to a sage for some clarity. I understand the desire to seek advice, and I do not want to avoid the client's genuine longing for direction. I have tried to change the way I think of giving advice and see it as more of a sort of guidance. This guidance looks less like standing out in front of the client and saying, "Come this way. Do it this way." Instead, I think of standing close behind the client, guiding them along their path while they walk forward on their own. I imagine whispering in their ear, not saying "turn left" or "turn right" because that might foster dependence. Instead, I whisper something more like, "There is a cross-roads ahead. What do you think you should do up there?"

Talking about advice-giving

It can help to be explicit with the client about what you do when it comes to giving advice. Let them know how you handle that aspect of your work. If you say, "I don't give advice," it might shut down a potential process. Instead, maybe you can say, "I am going to go beyond advice and help you find your own answers," or something like that. You might also empathize and talk about the process, saying, "I know you want advice, and I have some thoughts and ideas for you, yet I do not want to just stop at giving you advice. I want to help empower you to not only figure out what to do in this situation, but how to learn and grow from it and feel empowered the next time you are in a situation like this."

Here you might explain your rationale for why you do not give advice. There is a good reason. It is not just that you want to prevent advising the client in the wrong way and have them get mad at you. It is also that you would not necessarily know what is best for them. You might not have all the answers. Instead, you want to better understand the problem and help the client access their own native wisdom. Usually, there is something blocking their access to their wisdom, and you might help remove the constraints to them finding their own answers. Often the constraint is emotional. The emotional part of the brain is aroused, and they are unable to access their wisdom. In these moments, our job is to help soothe and calm them down, and then maybe the client's wise mind can come back online, and they can look at the problem together with you.

It is difficult when a client who has not historically been able to trust that their own wisdom will get them through tough times continues to be emotionally distressed at situations in their life. In those situations, a co-dependency can pull on you as the therapist, and you might be more susceptible to dispensing advice with the hope that it will help them feel less upset. When a client becomes dependent on you to tell them what to do, you can instead shift toward comforting and soothing their emotions and then help build up their confidence. You can remind them of times they figured out past problems or weathered past storms in their life. Reminding them that they have the capacity to figure it out and that you are there to figure it out with them can be all that they need to find their way.

Accessing deeper understanding

Any investigation into why we behave a certain way has to start with compassion. We have to convey to the client that we truly have compassion for why they are the way they are. We have to let them know that we get it. Giving the client a sense that we understand them and can relate to their experience is really a key foundational element to making therapy work.

For a client that feels reckless and wants your advice about how to be more in control of her life, you could directly say to her, "I hear that you feel out of control. Control gets a bad rap. We need to feel in control for love to get in. You cannot have things be out of control in your life." We could connect it to early experiences. "You told me in the past that when you were four and your parents divorced, everything felt out of control and you started throwing temper tantrums. Your emotions would take over and it was hard to receive any sort of help." Maybe then the client maps out a sense of herself so that we go more internal. Her request for advice about how to feel in control becomes a doorway to deeper work. That is the art of our work: to take the dilemma the client presents and, rather than getting caught up in advice, move into the deeper work of personal healing.

Guidance as advice

How do you get your client onto a path of looking inside themselves and growing personally when they keep asking for your advice? For example, what if a client says to you, "I think my partner is cheating on me, and

I saw some weird text messages. What should I do?" Do you give advice or not? Probably not. Yet what if the advice in this situation sounded like, "Okay, what if you just slow down? Let us look more closely at what might be going on here and talk with your partner." While the client might want advice about what to do about their potentially cheating partner, they really need more guidance from you as the therapist on how to slow down. When somebody asks you, "What should I do?" you might guide them to slow down and think through their options. In this example, do they want to talk to their partner? Do they want to be confrontational or not? They could think through the positives and negatives of how to respond. Your role is to help them become more organized.

What if a client came in and said, "My spouse just came to me and said she wants a divorce. My whole world is falling apart. What do I do?" It would feel really painful for the client if they heard, "Well, it is not really my job to tell you what to do. You need to find your own wisdom on this. What is getting in the way of you knowing what to do here?" That would be really unhelpful and frustrating for the client. Instead, we need to help them think through their options for handling this troubling situation.

It can be tempting to give advice. We do have wisdom and experience from being on the inside of many people's lives, and from that, we start to see what works for people. If you have walked couples through separation or telling their children about their divorce, or worked with a client while their partner was being unfaithful, then you have seen a little bit of what works for people to navigate those situations. Perhaps you have also read studies on what is typical in these life events and have a more keen sense of appropriate and effective ways for people to manage them. You might have valuable information that the client needs, and it may be an important time in their lives when you are not necessarily telling them what to do with their lives. Rather, you are advising them, consulting in a way, on potential directions they could move.

We are not interested in the content of the drama of people's lives. Instead, we are interested in their process of experiencing their life. We want to know how they cope and if they are finding adaptive ways of managing the struggles of life. We want to make sure that they are growing personally and developing social and emotional skills to be more effective in their lives. Being overly concerned with advice-giving interrupts the process of a client's learning and growing. Our real job is to help people cope better and develop themselves personally and relationally. The presenting problem is just the catalyst for this sort of growth. It is the opportunity to take somebody on a journey into themselves. If you have been on a journey with your clients, then you have gone through their life experiences and gotten to the other side with them. What was more important than advice-giving was being with them through it. Often relationship distress or something falling apart in the client's life will send them running into counseling. Our job, then, is to stabilize them first and then help them grow and develop.

Guiding change and transformation

Clients want to see evidence that therapy is working. Yet change is not always easy to measure. With therapy, the process is not always so tangible. Measuring change often depends on the presenting problem, and we might be able to note progress when the client reports a noticeable feeling that is different for them in their life. We could work with them to measure the change when it comes to new feelings or for them to notice a different thought pattern. We could track whether the client is reporting more self-awareness or freedom to make different behavioral choices. Just because a client keeps coming back to session does not necessarily mean the treatment is working. If they come back and say they did something different or showed up in new ways in their relationships, that may be measurable. When a client says, "I don't know what it was about this week, but it was way more peaceful at home. I noticed myself not as triggered," that is music to the ears of the therapist listening for change.

If you have been hiking up a mountain or driving up a hill, you usually do not realize how much you have climbed until you look out the rearview mirror or you stop and turn around to take in the view. Therapy is like a mountain without a top. There is always more work to be done. There is always more growth to be had. We may not know where we are on that path of growth until we stop and look down the mountain to see where we came from. We need to stop at times in therapy and review the progress that has been made. For if we don't, it will always feel like an endless climb.

I talked recently with a couple about their progress. We stopped and saw the change that they had made in just a couple of sessions. There is, of course, much more for them to work on beyond a few sessions, yet I wanted them to be aware of the changes that they already had made. This was not only for them to acknowledge the work that they had done but also to give them hope that they could make ongoing changes into the future in places that they thought might never be changed. This couple was split. One of the partners was saying that there was still a lot to do until the relationship felt better. The other was questioning why they need to keep coming to session if they had already made the improvements they had in those first few sessions. The happy medium for them was for us to consider that they had reached a base camp. We knew that we had made some progress and we should relish in it. We also needed to rid ourselves of any illusion that we were at the top of the mountain.

Sometimes when we reach a base camp in therapy, it is *not* useful to keep climbing. We ought to stop and acclimatize before making the next ascent. It is useful for some people to stop therapy and take in the new level of awareness that they have achieved. Having a built-in process for reviewing can help the client (and the therapist) track progress. We should regularly be measuring the changes that have occurred over time. Sometimes a motivated client will know that the progress is good but that they still have not cleared the tree line to get the amazing view. They know that they need to keep coming to therapy to achieve their personal goals. For others, it is really demoralizing if they keep coming to therapy but are not seeing much change. They see themselves repeating unhealthy patterns and do not know how to change. For these clients, it feels like they are still at the bottom of the mountain. Why would they keep going if months of therapy do not change the view? For these clients, they need more than change. They need transformation.

Being in the business of helping people transform is really a big undertaking. It is much bigger than causing change because, as the saying goes, "the more things change, the more they stay the same." While we want noticeable *change*, for some clients, change would not be very satisfying because they have yet to *transform*. For instance, if someone is depressed, we might help them change their behaviors so that they are more connected and less alone. That would be helping them change the context in which the problem exists. Their depression may still be there, but perhaps the person learns how to not get caught up in shame and blame and isolate themselves and instead find ways of being close to others. Maybe their relationships are a bit kinder, and they learn how to communicate with others more effectively. Sometimes that change in behavior and perspective might make all the difference and is all that is needed for that person.

Others might need more. They might need to transform their depression into something more empowering and life-affirming. These clients might be able to go into the depths of themselves and emerge someone entirely new. Our job is to find what is possible and help the client access the most of what they can get from therapy. We can see transformation available for everyone who comes through our doors. We can be keenly aware of the best of what therapy can do and help each client get there. If you know the potential of therapy, but there is not very much progress, then it will not feel satisfying. As mentioned earlier, it is like having a five-speed sports car and going slowly in second gear. You know what is possible with this process and that we could really open things up. By seeing you, the client could become a whole new person, confront their shadow, and learn new ways of relating. Yet if there is not much progress, then you are just cruising around in second gear. Maybe slow progress is needed sometimes, and at least the client is going somewhere, even if it is slowly. While it might be frustrating for you to move along so slowly with the therapeutic process, at least they are engaged. The key is to gauge how much change or transformation is even available at that moment and adjust your approach accordingly.

We need to define what causes people to change and what causes people to transform. There may be many things, yet unfortunately, quite often, it is pain that causes people to transform. When something is painful enough, we would do anything to transform it, so the pain stops. For a client who struggles in relationships, for instance, repetitive, painful patterns might be enough for them to transform. If they keep experiencing similar challenges, it could be so painful for the client that they might become motivated to change. By losing everything, they might become willing to look more closely at how they have been and start examining how they might be different in relationships. This would be the moment to work toward transformation in therapy. Timing is everything, and if you had tried to get the client to transform before, they might have been resistant. Yet when things fall apart, there might be an opportunity to get the therapy process unstuck.

Compassionate confrontation is key when the client is stuck. When we sense that transformation is not feasible, we may want to level with them. You could say something like, "I do not think you are ready to do this yet, but if you were to be less controlling in your relationship, I think you would be in less pain. It is less about this relationship and more about your need to transform your self-esteem. Your self-talk is so negative. If you are not really willing to take that on and be kind to yourself, then I do not know how much we are going to be able to do right now. You are going to keep coming in and reporting how things feel out of control and that your spouse is such a jerk. We are not going to see change until you start to look inside yourself and develop a kinder way of relating to yourself."

It is a really powerful role that we hold for people. We want to err on the side of being safe and cautious, not telling our clients exactly how to live their lives. Instead, we can see ourselves as helping guide people toward their better selves. If you keep advice at bay and instead focus on opportunities for transformation, your clients will thank you in the end.

16

HOW MUCH IS A SESSION WORTH?

This chapter discusses the financial realities of working in the mental health field. Getting clear about the value of therapy sessions and seeing how our time can be priceless helps clinicians ground their practice in financial health. How does a client know the value of therapy when clinical progress is often unclear? We need to be solid in knowing our value and make sure we are compensated properly based on experience. Doing so can provide a strong basis for effective therapy. If a therapist is charging too much, then they will likely feel pressure to perform clinically. If they are undercompensated then that might impact their clinical work as well. This chapter addresses the importance of managing the financial aspect of one's clinical practice well so that there is a proper framework for ongoing care.

The price of therapy

Clients and therapists alike can feel ambivalent about the financial aspects of therapy. Even though they really value the services they receive, clients may feel like the therapist only cares about them because the client

DOI: 10.4324/9781003283164-17

is paying for sessions. On the other hand, therapists might love what they do and would do it for free if they could, but at the same time need to make a living and feel underpaid for their services. It's a complicated process, and we need to think progressively about how we handle money in therapy rather than get caught in old, predictable traps when it comes to providing care for service.

By its very nature, the service we offer, providing support and care for others, is confused by money being involved. People typically associate a caring relationship with someone who is willing to give freely of themselves because they are innately concerned. When we attach a fee to the service, then we add a stipulation. If you don't pay for my time, then I won't provide the service. It might be easier if we were selling goods such as clothing, apparel, or small appliances. The costs associated with a customer receiving the product would be less complicated. It is understood that they have to pay to get the merchandise. It is a business selling the product, after all. Yet since we provide counseling services, there is much more complexity. Clients might not see what we do as a business in and of itself. Because of this, we must be ready to grapple with the nuances involved in collecting fee for services.

Whether we are compensated by a larger organization such as an agency, hospital, or school, or if we are in a private or group practice where we are paid directly by the client or their insurance, we must be conscious of how money impacts therapy. It can be difficult to put a price on therapy because the outcomes are usually ambiguous. If I go to the barber or hairstylist for their services, I can see that they cut, styled, or colored my hair. If I go to the dentist, I can feel that they cleaned my teeth. Yet, with therapy, it can be difficult for the client to feel that they are getting something of value. I would never negotiate fee with my barber or dentist, yet it can be a customary part of the practice of therapy to discuss fees and consider lowering them to meet the needs of the client.

It is not that our services are less valuable than the stylist's or dentist's. It is just that they are harder to measure. How does a client know that they got what they paid for? Perhaps if their symptoms ease or if they find new coping strategies, they might say that therapy was worth the fee. Yet typically, it is hard to know when therapy is complete. We might see the process as a mountain without a top. There are endless areas to work on in therapy, and we may never reach the summit. There are basecamps along the way where one might pause in their process of personal growth, but they may never be ultimately finished with the climb. Furthermore, unlike cutting hair or cleaning teeth, the work of therapy is oftentimes invisible. It happens on the inside, and clients may not clearly identify the changes happening within. Because of this, the price of therapy is often difficult to gauge.

How much is a session worth?

Essentially, a client pays for your presence. Their fee is for the 50 minutes of your time during which you are expected to be deeply present with them. Your time, and your ability to be impactful during that time, is where the value lies. Your goal is to use that time to create the greatest impact and make that session worthwhile. When a client comes to session they are usually in pain of some sort. They want relief from the pain, and our job is to convey to them that going through the process of therapy is worth it and that they will find relief from their pain. We hope that they will trust us to go on a journey of personal growth and that there will be results in the end. If, ultimately, the client has a tremendous, life-changing breakthrough during session, then how could one put a price tag on that? Even though we know that it can take months or years to get to that sort of breakthrough, all of the time and resources spent would be worth it if the client's life changed for the better.

Even though this journey may be priceless, we still must determine how much our time and presence are worth and set our fee accordingly. The fee for a session is a delicate thing. We need to carefully consider what our time is worth and what can the client pay for that time. If you overcharge a client, then it can lead to clinical pressure. If you charge too little, then you might feel undervalued. Finding the right fee that honors your experience but fits within a realistic budget for the client would be the ideal setup for clinical balance and success.

When I was a new professional, right out of graduate school working as a post-graduate clinical fellow, the fee for service caused me undue pressure. Prior to the fellowship, while working in the training clinic as a student, the fee that the clients paid was on a sliding scale, 20 dollars and under. Some paid one dollar per session, and I didn't see any of that fee because I was a student in training. After graduating one day, having been charging 20 dollars and under, the next day, when the fellowship started, I began charging 90 dollars per session. In one day, my fee jumped so much that I began to panic. I felt like I had to make things happen in session so that the clients got their money's worth. In each session, I would throw hypothesis and theory at the client, trying everything I could to make the meeting impactful. Because of this pressure, I ended up being less effective than if I had sat back and trusted the process as I was more easily able to do as a trainee in the clinic with a lower client fee.

What was really underneath this frantic approach to therapy was that I did not feel worth 90 dollars an hour. My presence and experience did not seem to me to warrant that high of a fee. To make matters more complicated, a few months into my fellowship, I was referred a client who worked as a higher-level executive and wanted to work with a male therapist. The referring therapist thought I would be a good fit, and the client was okay seeing a fellow. We ended up having a good rapport, and he attended regularly for over a year. Over time I started to feel settled enough to be worth the fee he was paying. When this client casually disclosed the amount of his year-end bonus, and when I realized that it was more than twice what I was making in salary, I felt incredibly undervalued. While I still didn't feel worth the 90 dollar an hour fee, it also didn't feel right to be earning such a low income compared to my client. I think that I was still able to do effective therapy with him, but money and worth were always in the room with us when we met.

Balancing what we love with what we earn

After that fellowship, I realized that I had some work to do about the financial aspect of therapy. I needed to find a way to feel worth the client's fee while also generate appropriate income to make a living as a clinician. While I loved where I was working post-fellowship, enjoying the security of building my practice within a larger institution, I had a painful realization when I realized that my rate of compensation was only 20 percent of what I charged the client per session. Recognizing that I was compensated such a low percentage of the client fee made me take stock in how I could better balance the work that I love with making a sustainable living.

Each therapist needs to figure out for themselves the right balance between doing what they love and making a living. If you love your clients but feel undervalued and don't enjoy where you work, then it might not be a sustainable situation. If you are making a lot per session but work long late hours, then you might be susceptible to burnout. Making sure that you are compensated fairly while also doing what you love in an environment that feels healthy is a recipe for a long, fulfilling career. That sort of balance may also reflect positively on your clinical work. While we are all professionals and likely will do good clinical work even if we are not in the best work environments, there is added benefit in working somewhere where we feel valued. There is a parallel process when the therapist feels cared for and appreciated by their employer, and it gets reflected clinically. The clients feel cared for and valued when the therapist does too.

This parallel process is much like the one between supervisor and supervisee. Something gets transmitted from the larger system to the one being cared for. Water runs downhill, as it were. If the employing organization is transparent and solid in how it cares for and compensates it's staff, then there is more likelihood that the clients seen by those staff members will feel cared for as well. Caring for the staff is the best quality assurance that an organization can do.

Healthy finances and accounts receivable

It is also important as therapists that we take care of all of the financial details between us and our clients. If we are not comfortable talking about our fees and making them explicit, then it can cause imbalances in the therapeutic framework. Having numerous clients who fail to pay their bill on time or who run balances can be a sign that we are not giving enough attention to the financial part of the therapeutic relationship. While the relationship is grounded in care, it is also a business agreement. We agree to provide the service, and the client agrees to pay their bill. Having a clear discussion about these expectations upfront in the first session, including what your cancellation policy is, can help set expectations. Yet if these conversations are not had, and we need to address a balance on the client's account later in the course of therapy for, say, a cancellation with charge, then the client might feel blindsided if they were unaware of your policy. In those moments, the care that is implicit in the relationship can become questioned.

I have seen very talented therapists lose clients because they did not handle finances with their clients in a healthy way. Some were either too casual about the business side of the therapeutic relationship, or others were too strict and overly formal about money. There needs to be a balanced, relaxed way to incorporate the financial aspect of the therapist–client relationship so that it is naturally embedded into what we do. Without that sort of approach, conversations about money can ruin an otherwise productive course of therapy. Clients can feel embarrassed about a bill that they owe, or they can feel taken advantage of or unfairly treated if it seems that the therapist is just focused on money. Being able to have clear conversations with clients about money can help the therapeutic relationship. The expectations just need to be clear.

While clients can feel mistreated by the therapist for improper management of finances, therapists can feel devalued when the client does not pay their bill. If clients do not honor their side of the therapeutic agreement, then we can become resentful in ways that compromise the unconditional positive regard we are taught to hold. Feelings about money can be charged, and they can leak into sessions in ways that we are not always fully aware of. Clients might resent having to pay for someone to listen to them, and we might feel upset about the low value put on our time. Rather than becoming reactive or defensive about money and therapy, we must sew up the financial piece so that it works for everyone involved.

17

ATTENTION, MERGING, AND GUILT: HOW TO STAY BALANCED AS A THERAPIST

In this chapter, we cover how to manage our own attention in the room, what to do when we merge with clients, and how to not carry our clients with us. We also look at how guilt plays a role in caring for others and how to say balanced.

Paying attention and understanding worry

A friend of mine has adult attention deficit disorder (ADD). We were at the baseball game a little while back, talking and watching the game. We were both simultaneously managing the game and our conversation at the same time, yet he was also listening to the conversation going on in the row behind us and a couple of seats down.

"Can you believe what these people are saying behind us?" he asked. He was not just tracking the baseball game and our talk but also following the conversation of the people who were a few seats away. This was a clear illustration to me that ADD is not an *attention* issue but a *filtering* issue.

DOI: 10.4324/9781003283164-18

There was extra information that my friend with ADD was processing in that moment and also on a regular basis.

If you think about it, you are constantly processing information. Your body is handling so much stimuli and so much information moment to moment that you have learned to filter out a lot of it and focus on a particular experience in front of you. Because of this, our minds stop experiencing the world as something new every day. If you had just pure sensory experiences every day, it would be too much. For somebody with ADD, perhaps we can honor the amount of stimulus and input their mind and body are taking in and consider that they are not filtering it very well.

For my friend at the baseball game, if something really important was happening on the field, then he probably would have changed up how he integrated the information. I doubt with a home run, he would have still been tracking everything, as the homer would have drawn in more of his attention. Similarly, if you are driving from one point to another, there are, of course, a lot of things going on inside every house, inside every store, and in the streets along your way. You are not going to stop and look in every window of every home and store on your way home. You would never get home at that rate. You have to block out some of that information to get home. We all have to do that every day in order to socialize.

What draws your attention?

As the clinician in the room, where do you put your attention? There are a number of stimuli in the clinical room when you are working with a client – maybe not as much as if you were at a crowded baseball game, but a lot. Your attention could be on the client, or it could be on you. It could be on the ideas, the words, the feelings going on, or it could be on the clock, the temperature in the room, your tummy that hurts, or the fight you had last night with your partner. Where do you notice your attention tends to go when you are with clients?

Hopefully, your attention is on more than just words. There is way more going on in the room than what is being said. By recognizing that there is more to attend to than what's being spoken, you are able to gather more information, more data, that might inform your strategizing and thinking about the case. You would not say to the client, "I notice you are wearing new shoes today," or "As a couple you are sitting so far apart. I'm just noticing that." Instead, you use that information to form some sort of hypothesis about the client. All the nonverbal information that you notice in the room goes into your thinking. Some of the nonverbal data is not even tangible. It is just something you feel in the subtext. Paying attention to that is part of the work.

If you can expand your attention so that it is not fixated on the client or what is being said, you allow yourself to be more open to pertinent case material. You have to pay attention to where you are putting your attention, otherwise, you might run on autopilot and become either narrowly focused or zoned out. If you pay too much attention to the client and not enough to yourself and your own thoughts and feelings, then you might become de-selfed in a way. If you are preoccupied with your own mind, then you might not tune in enough your client. The key is to find balance, a bifurcated approach in which part of your attention is on the content of the session, and another part is on the process and the nonverbals. This can help you stay attuned to your client yet open to other stimuli.

Like my friend at the baseball game, we need our perception to be unfiltered so that we can take in everything that shows up in a therapy session, both within the client and within ourselves. We also want to be able to focus our attention in a laser-like way on the work at hand. If a client starts sharing a traumatic experience, we want to be able to hone our attention onto the trauma work so that we do not miss anything. Being able to tune in and out like a satellite dish receiving various signals but dialing into the needed station helps keep the therapeutic process on track.

Separating yourself from your client

If your attention in session is so keyed in that you have strong mirroring somatic experiences or feel what your client is feeling, it is even more important to track where you put your attention and awareness. An empathic clinician may feel deeply what the client is feeling and may not know who is who and what is what. The empathic therapist's central nervous system gets thrown off in session, and it may have nothing to do with what is happening inside of them but instead entirely from the client. It can be difficult to tell.

How can we discern if what we are feeling or sensing is our own or if it is coming from our clients? Perhaps what is throwing the therapist off is their own countertransference. Or maybe it has to do with the struggles in their personal life. We need to be able to tell whose psychological energy is whose and to make out whose feelings are whose. When it gets jumbled up, it is very difficult to know where thoughts and feelings are coming from. You might start to have similar thoughts and feelings as your client without recognizing it at first. There can be a contagion effect from working closely with your clients.

Ideally, you are over here in your therapy chair, and your client is over there on the couch. The two of you can connect because you are discrete entities. It is easier to be close to someone else when there is this sort of clarity. I can get close to someone else because I do not get mixed in with them. There is a sort of codependence when I am mixed in with them. It becomes hard for me to be close because I have to move away at some point to maintain my sense of self. At that point, I cannot see clearly because the other person is inside of me, and I am inside of the other person. This is not intimacy. This is like two young lovers just charging into each other because it feels so good to merge.

You really have to be careful as an empathic clinician not to merge with your client. Joining is one thing, merging is another. If you hold somebody else's suffering inside of you, it feels like poison. You cannot metabolize it. Most therapists are walking around filled in and mixed up with their clients' suffering. No wonder they get compassion fatigue or burnout!

I had an experience earlier in my career in which I worked with a client who was feeling low self-esteem. He felt like he was not good enough and that he was alone in life. He was wondering what the use was in living. We did some good work one session in which we were very connected, and I felt that I was supporting him. It was my last session of the day, and after it ended, I did my notes and went home. I was walking back to my place, musing about how tough of a day it was. I wondered to myself whether or not I even made a difference. I questioned if I was even good at this. I wondered who I even have to talk to about all of this. I felt really alone and down about myself. I wondered what the use was in even trying.

Then I recognized that I was feeling exactly what the last client of the day was feeling. It seemed like I was feeling these things because it was my thoughts and bodily sensations, yet I was actually carrying what my client was feeling and had not properly separated from him at the end of the day. You could say I had injected him into me. From an energetic standpoint, I had absorbed him and was carrying him. Doing so was not serving him, and it certainly did not serve me either. This moment when I recognized that I had not yet separated out from him really helped me. It allowed me to get back to myself and to recognize that I was okay.

You have to be really careful if you are an empathic person because if you can feel what is going on with people, you can lose yourself in them. Becoming aware of getting mixed in on a subtle level with your clients can be a really big first step toward discernment. Discernment helps prevent burnout. To be discerning, it would help to cleanse yourself of the sessions you have each day. You must find a way to shake them off somehow and not carry them around with you after you leave the office.

There are many ways you can do this. Find a way to wring yourself out like a sponge. You could use creative visualization and imagine that what you are holding is leaving you. You could do an activity that shakes the day of sessions off of you such as exercising, yoga, or cooking. Finding something that helps you feel better is a good step. Some therapists just go and drink, but that does not really provide the needed discernment. It is just a way of numbing out. Instead, you need something holistic to help you leave your clients at the office, to send the sessions out of you, perhaps down, down into the Earth, or out into space. Let the sessions go and connect with yourself so that you are clearer for the next day.

Guilt, care, and worry

As caring therapists, we need to be especially careful about guilt. It can compel us to conduct ourselves in ways that are not always the most therapeutic. Guilt might cause us to compromise our boundaries in the hopes of being loving and caring. Guilt is a control. It controls our free will and prevents us from living life fully and being well. It grabs us by the head and keeps us from being free to move on to the next thing in life. Guilt says, "If you cared, then you would …" It makes us question ourselves.

If you had a session with a client who was alone and suffering, and then you left to go have a joyous night out with loved ones, guilt might tell you that you do not really care about that client's suffering. It would make you feel bad for having a joyous night while your client struggles alone. How can you enjoy life when others you care about suffer? This is an impulse of most therapists who work closely with their clients, yet it is not sustainable to forgo one's life for the sake of honoring another's pain.

Perhaps a way that we can truly be of service to others is to not lose our light and not dim our life, even in the presence of someone who is stuck and suffering. Obviously, we should not gloat, rub it in, or tell them about what a joyous weekend we had while they complain of suffering alone. If they are stuck in a bad place, it does not help for you to be stuck there with them. Just as high tide raises all boats, if you maintain your optimism, it might allow others to find some hope amidst their struggles.

With guilt, I encourage you to take it on piece by piece. Try forgetting about your client just for a little bit after the session and see what happens. Maybe you say to yourself, "Okay, I will worry about them tonight, but for my commute home, I am not going to think about them." And then just see what happens. Does the time not worrying about your client actually mean that you care less? Did the client suffer more because you did not worry about them for an hour? Just try a little bit here and there to find some space away from thinking about your client. Perhaps these little breaks can help you slip out of the control of guilt that tells you about how lousy we are as a therapist.

In an extreme example, such as when a client is suicidal, it would not be clinically sound to be worry-free and forget your clients. Your worry sometimes alerts you to take steps that help protect the client. You would not just dismiss your worry in those instances. When a client is suffering emotionally or stuck in bad relationship patterns but is not in distress, your excessive worry outside of session does no additional good.

There is a difference between love and worry, and when we get those confused, burnout often happens. A parent may say to a child, "I am just so worried about you," which to the parent means I love you. Yet there is actually a big difference between worrying about a person and loving them. When you are worried for them, you are carrying them. And when you are loving them, you are freeing them. The child may say back to the parent, "Please do not give me your worry. Give me your love instead!"

Worrying when we feel unhelpful

If you have a sense of not being effective with your client, then your worry might go up. You might unconsciously say to yourself, "Well at least I am being neurotic about the case. I must really care!" Worrying about a client acts as a substitute for not knowing what to do with the case.

I had a couples counseling case where we had a great second session, and then in the third session, they said their relationship was over. I felt very discouraged and like I did not actually help them. That session ended on a low note, with them saying they were going to take a break from each other and would let me know about coming back to therapy. While I felt like I did the best I could, considering I was just getting to know the case, I still spent the rest of the evening and many times throughout the week worrying about this couple and thinking about them. Instead of getting consultation about how to be more effective with this case, I just worried.

Guilt whispers in our ears in these vulnerable moments, saying, "If you really care, you should worry, because then it will feel like you are actually doing something." This obviously is not helpful. Instead, we need to be okay with not doing anything in these moments that feel helpless. We need to be okay with trying our best to be there for our clients. We could clarify and connect with our theory of change and start to embody it. We can deepen our understanding of how people really heal and grow and then get ourselves ready for the next day of being with other human beings, our clients, that need our deep care.

18

ANXIETY IS LIKE A HAND WITHOUT FINGERS

In this chapter, we discuss when and how to recommend resources to clients such as books or podcasts and what might prompt those resource recommendations. We also explore how to take those recommendations deeper and encourage clients to go further into themselves. We look at what shadow work looks like and how to use metaphors more effectively.

Recommending resources to clients

It is important to get clear about when and in what ways you recommend resources to clients. Whether it is a book, podcast, television show, YouTube video, seminar, or recommendation for a therapy group, those extra resources can make a difference. One consideration is that you should know the resource first. Do you subscribe to the content and think it would be valuable? If a client asks if you know of a book about a topic, and you have only heard of that book, then it may not necessarily

DOI: 10.4324/9781003283164-19

be a good referral source because you do not really know the content through and through.

The second consideration is how you frame your recommendation. You would not just offer a recommendation unless there was some context for it. For example, you could say, "We have been talking about codependency for a while and I think that we agree that it is a place where you are stuck. 50-minute sessions get us somewhere, but would you be open to doing more work on this and read about co-dependency to get more information? If so, there is a book I think might be good for you. Please do not take everything in this book as doctrine, but it may be a good place to start getting more information on codependency."

This sort of framing gives context for why you are recommending a resource. It allows the client to integrate their reading or viewing into the framework of therapy with you. If a client asks you for a recommendation on a particular topic, and you do not have one, then it is okay to tell them that you will check around and see what you can find. It is okay for them to see you as not having that resource on tap. They may value that you are willing to do the research to find a book. If you know of a book but do not necessarily know the book's contents, then say that you have heard of it or that colleagues have recommended this book but that you are not guaranteeing it.

There can be a frame in which we encourage our clients to direct their own learning. There are a lot of resources available for people for personal growth and development, whereas, in the distant past, they may have been harder to find. It might be more effective to free your client to go find resources themselves. They can do a deeper dive into topics of interest to them and do their own research on personal growth and development in order to be more fully nourished in certain areas.

Therapy with you can be like a Michelin-starred fine dining restaurant where clients get a small taste of an incredible bite of information. They do not need overflowing bowls of pasta all at once. Sometimes less is more with a client, and they can do more healing and growth work outside of session. It is okay if we cannot do everything for the client and have every answer for them. Maybe just a little bit of something nourishing in session with you can cause a difference for them and be transformative.

We just want to make sure that we are not recommending resources as a defense against feeling ineffective, not knowing about a particular topic, or not being able to help the client completely. Often our recommendation is exactly what the client needs. Sometimes a well-timed worksheet, workbook, activity, or homework is perfectly called for. Yet other times, we might recommend a resource as a defense against muddling through the work with them in session. It is important for us to know when we are using external resources as a way of supplementing our work and when we are fleeing a sense of being out of our depths with the presenting problem.

If we are stuck and do not know how to say exactly what we want to say to a client because we are worried that it might hurt their feelings, or they might become reactive, then we may also flee to a book or podcast as a more palatable recommendation. While this can help in the short term, we might also want to look at why we cannot bring the needed interaction into session. Is there a sense that if we were direct with the client that it would not be well received? If so, then we could track what stymies us such that we feel we need to bring in some external resource.

Doing shadow work with clients

When we are stymied and reflexively reach for external resources to support our work, we ought to instead consider going deeper with the work. Helping clients look within at the parts of them that they are afraid of can take courage on our parts, but it can make all the difference. It is something that we call shadow work. These shadowy areas are the parts of clients that cause them a lot of distress and are aspects of their lives that they spend a lot of time privately thinking about. They let us into the inner recesses of their psyche when they share their shadow material with us. These are the ego-dystonic aspects of the client that are not integrated into their egoic sense of self. Our work is to try to make these aspects more ego-syntonic so that those parts of the self can be somehow integrated into their conceptualization of who they are.

Once a client asked me in session, "If I'm a creative person and a caring mother, then how is it that I also have these strange, dark fantasies of running off to another country with my coworker?" She was referring to how she fixated on this coworker and what he represented to her. More encouragingly, when it came to our therapy, she was wondering how both of these aspects of herself (creative, caring mother and obsessed, fixated escapist) exist within her. She was describing the human struggle of having seemingly disjointed aspects of who we are and longing to find a way to integrate these various aspects into our self-conceptualization.

If you have a client who has some rigidity around their sense of self, where they cannot accept being paradoxical in nature and instead insist on being one way or another, then you have your work cut out for you. You might have to move more slowly in therapy so that the client can start sharing any parts of themselves they are ashamed of with you. If a client feels that getting in touch with these shadow aspects of self that they will become overtaken, then we want to approach it carefully and maybe even indirectly. It is almost as if we want to look at the shadow together with our clients out of the corner of our mind's eye. We could reference that there is this thing over there that we want to gather some surveillance data about. We can imagine looking through a one-way mirror to a room where this shadow thing exists so we can safely start relating to it. In this way, the client might be able to observe aspects of who they are without fearing being overrun, but also without distancing themselves from who they are. A Narrative Therapy approach works well here.

One aspect of the therapeutic relationship is to try to create some normalization around the client's experience. We usually want to convey that what the client is experiencing is pretty typical to the human experience. Even though it may not be *healthy*, the client's experience might be *common*. Normalizing the experience can help them approach and integrate the shadow aspects of themselves. We want to let the client know that what they are going through is something that we might have experienced ourselves or witnessed in a previous client. In other words, in our sessions, we are saying, "You are not alone in this experience." In sharing this, the client can start to relate to themselves differently.

Typically, the way that the client relates to their shadow is probably not as healthy as it could be. It is likely a punitive, critical relationship that prevents their shadow from evolving and transforming. The client needs not to just *change* their shadow self, but to *transform* it into something that feels good for them. In order to do that transformative work, there needs to be a foundation of health. There needs to be some normalization, some compassion, and some acceptance. We must keep in mind that acceptance for the shadow is different than permission. Just because we accept that we do shadowy things does not mean that we are giving ourselves permission to keep doing it. Once we get there, to a place of acceptance, then some transformation and healing can occur.

Integrating client's sense of self

Looking at our shadow is challenging. It is scary to look at ourselves in general, and when we approach our more shameful aspects, it can be even more difficult. A client may not even want to look at themselves at all, but our goal as compassionately confrontational clinicians is to make it safe enough for them to look at their shadow. For instance, we might want a client to really be in touch with their anxiety rather than verbally describing it. We can first ask them to externalize the anxiety as if we are looking at it together through a one-way mirror so that they can safely see this aspect of who they are. The externalizing is the first part, which makes it a little safer to look. Then we want to move toward integrating what they observe about themselves into their self-concept.

The goal is to integrate the shadow aspect while also understanding how it got split off in the first place. We want to try understand how the client got shut down previously in their life. What messages came in that made the client the way that they are? Was there familial or social conditioning that told the client to stay muted or repressed? Did they have to shut down in order to survive? We know that if we shut down or shut off a part of ourselves, it will often leak out sideways or manifest itself in some other way. Getting the client to see this for themselves can go a long way toward their personal growth and toward a deeper feeling of an integration of who they are.

For instance, when asked to view her anxiety through a one-way mirror, one client shared with her therapist that she saw it as a hand without fingers. It was there trying to hold onto the world and connect but couldn't do anything because it lacked grip. This personified her anxiety. The therapist was then able to get the client to relate to her fingerless hand of anxiety in new ways. She was able to help her have compassion for this aspect of herself that longed to connect in any real and significant way and made a connection to how this paralyzed part of herself was acting out through having an affair.

The client was more readily able to see that she may likely have been splitting off an aspect of herself into the extramarital relationship. It was easier for her to see that the affair was probably a symptom of having felt like she could not bring a more alive, creative aspect of herself into her marital life. Whether it is social conditioning, patriarchy, the marriage, family of origin, or the client's own beliefs about parenthood and self-sacrifice, powerful forces might be enacting on our clients that cause them to believe that vital elements of who they are have to go away once they are at a certain level of maturity or adulthood.

The notion of having to live it up in one's teens and 20s and then get serious starting in one's 30s could contribute to a recipe for repression, anxiety, and acting out. How many great people do we see brought down because they just cannot keep themselves from doing something racy or explicit, even if they had much to lose professionally and personally? Perhaps people in this situation feel like they have to squash a vital aspect of themselves in order to fit in. For clients like this, they may need a warning from you as the therapist. They may need to hear you express your concern for their imbalanced behavior and then help them find a way to integrate it into their core sense of self.

Taking a stand and helping a client find integration within themselves can be very powerful therapeutically. Using some externalization, normalization, and integration, little by little, they find a more connected way of being in the world.

19

THERAPY POSTURE: HOW TO ORIENT YOURSELF IN SESSION

This chapter examines how to orient ourselves in session with clients, focusing on how we set our mindset to be with clients. By learning to be grounded and see clearly, we open up new possibilities for managing emotions and finding wisdom. This chapter also discusses how to stay grounded in session and how to create a sense of safety for the client. It looks at how to step back from the content of sessions so that we can have more clarity about treatment goals and how a therapist can balance their wisdom and emotion to create a humane connection with their clients.

Being grounded

What is the most fundamental and essential quality that is needed for therapy? What is the one element that makes everything else possible? While listening deeply to our clients is certainly key, creating a sense of safety is probably the most crucial cornerstone for effective therapy and

DOI: 10.4324/9781003283164-20

is a common factor across most therapeutic modalities. We really cannot do much else without creating safety with our clients. Creating a safe space, a safe relationship with the client is something that we all sense is the core of our work, yet understanding how to go about helping others feel safe is a skill. Beyond assuring the client that the session is confidential, there are important ways that we can orient ourselves in session so that it generates a sense of safety.

One way to create safety is to be grounded. Actually, having a sense of feeling at home and safely grounded within your body is important to therapy. If the therapist feels safely embodied, the client has a chance to feel safe too. The mechanics of being grounded are just like it is with electricity. The grounding wire creates safety and prevents explosions. If you try to jump your car battery, you make sure that you have one cable grounded so that it does not short circuit. It is the same thing with us as humans. We need to be grounded in order to keep things from flaming out.

Conveying to the client that we are grounded sends a message that if things get emotionally chaotic in session that it is okay. This is especially important if you are working with more than one person in the room. Sessions can easily get chaotic in couple and family therapy, and clients need to know that you are a center of calmness. The hope is that you can be grounded and have feelings running through you all at the same time, much like how electric wires are always live but remain safely contained. Conceivably, you could have negative feelings and reactions toward your clients, and it could still be safe. You might be angry with them, you might have disdain for them, you might be turned off by them, yet if you are safe and grounded, it could still be therapeutic for the clients.

We need to be aware that the process of therapy usually does not feel inherently safe to people and differs from person to person based on their backgrounds. Looking inside oneself means we may find something we do not want to confront. When a client sits down with you, and you ask them how they are, in a way that can be threatening. Most likely, their previous experiences with being asked to express what is inside of themselves have not gone very well, particularly if they experienced invalidation when doing so in the past. Your background and identities might also cause the client to feel unsafe, threatened, or judged.

In fact, the biggest fear that your clients likely have about you is that you are judging them and what they say. They assume that you are saying one thing in session, but you are thinking something else. This is not really your fault, as your clients are probably used to people being inauthentic with them in their lives. If they feel that you are not authentic, then they are going to assume the worst, which is likely that on some level, you do not like them. Your posture in session can convey to the client that it might be more safe than what they are accustomed to when speaking with another human being. The way you express yourself, the tone of your voice, and your body language can send signals that you are a safe person to be with that knows how to hold space for others. Your posture can be consciously altered so that you are conscious of how you carry yourself, yet most of what generates authentic posture has more to do with how you place your awareness within your own body.

Step back to see clearly

Realistically, it is more probable that you are safe to be with, that you do indeed like your clients, and that you work to make sure you find ways to like them. There is, in all likelihood, much more going on within you in session than the client realizes. You might have strong reactions from your gut, powerful tugs at your heartstrings, and tons of ideas about what you want to say. There might be a range of reactions happening inside of you that might help inform your work, but it creates a lot of static that gets in the way of you seeing clearly. In order to see your client's situation more clearly, it might help to have less static coming from your gut, fewer impulses coming from your heart, and fewer ideas bouncing around in your mind.

It certainly might feel nice to practice from the heart, and it also might seem very real to practice from your gut. Practicing from your mind might also seem helpful. Those are all perfectly good places to practice from. Yet you are not going to see your clients as clearly as if you practice from a more neutral place that I like to call the center of your head.

The center of your head is just behind your eyes. It is a place within you where you can see and know. Rather than the wild and woolly place of the heart, or the intensity of the gut, the center of the head is a center of awareness that looks out into the world, into your life, and into the lives of others with clarity, compassion, and understanding. Different from the thinking mind, where ideas, hypotheses, and thoughts run wild, the center of the head is akin to a camera lens. You might look out on your life from the center of your head and get clear images or understanding about what is happening. It can be your seat of knowing as a therapist.

The center of your head could be a metaphorical place. Yet it also could literally be the part of your body that is right behind your eyes, near the pineal gland. You might have heard it called the third eye. It is an aspect of us that sees what is on the inside of ourselves and others. Our actual eyes see the physical world, while the third eye sees the metaphysical world. It sees beyond the physical. Talk therapy takes place beyond the physical, so it can help to be able to see clearly in this realm. Seeing clearly as a therapist is different from simply having thoughts or interventions. It is seeing what shows up as a picture in your mind's eye while you are in session and trusting in those images because they contain information that might address more deeply what is happening for your client.

You should certainly bring the theoretical training in your mind, the care in your heart, and the fire in your gut to session. Those are all vital aspects of practice. Those parts of you are where your therapeutic tools and your clinical style come from. Yet if you anchor yourself in the center of your head, then your sessions might feel more effortless. From the center of your head, you can listen to your mind, heart, and gut, but you will not be pulled by them into an ungrounded place. You will instead be gently seated in a more neutral center of awareness where you can also be in touch with inner self, looking at any pictures that show up in your mind's eye.

Dialing down the more intensely emotional parts of you and sitting in the center of your own head could change the way you practice so that you can see things more neutrally and have access to a sort of higher wisdom. While having your emotions dialed up in session can feel more intense and familiar, it has side effects. You might leave after a day of practicing from your heart or gut and feel exhausted. You might feel worried about the state of the world, need to numb out, or end up taking things out on those around you at home. Although it can feel like you gave it your all, it might not be the best thing to practice from your heart or gut. Certainly, there are some therapists who practice this way, and with every client, they are very wrapped up in the work. It just may not be very sustainable. It can be difficult to have a personal life being so wrapped up in clients that way. It might feel good because the therapist is wrapped up in the work and feels like they are making a difference, but they are going to be a puddle by the end of the week.

Hopefully, you are grounded and moored in a place within yourself where you are able to be with the client during whatever is going on in their life and act as a very wise and caring witness. Being a witness can be very healing. It provides neutral companionship while empowering the client to find their own answers to life's questions. If you notice, there is an aspect of yourself that is always witnessing what is going on in your life. That part is the doorway to what we might call your higher wisdom. This part of you does not get too caught up in the ups and downs of life. It watches with care and quietly offers insight and reassurance. Getting in touch with that part of ourselves helps us and also helps our clients because they feel reassured by it. Even if you have a strong reaction, thought or feeling in session and witness a client going through something challenging, you might also be in touch with a sense that they are eventually going to be okay.

Balancing wisdom and emotion

What is that perfect zone where we combine our wisdom, just enough emotion, plenty of insight and information, and fire from our belly? Where is that place that is safe and that has room for emotions and care? Finding it within yourself is a big undertaking and is the core of developing oneself as a clinician. It is the process of tuning your instrument so that seeing clients on a daily basis becomes effortless and enjoyable. You can learn clinical techniques and new methods of treatment, but without finding this sweet spot within yourself, you are left to practice in a way that might feel laborious and unnatural.

Our goal is to be human, commune with our clients, and care for them while not burning out in the process. It is a pretty lofty goal and a sacred undertaking that we have a chance to continually develop and refine. This sort of development as a clinician is not something that we learn in textbooks. Instead, it is through session after session with clients and through trying out different ways of being with them that we come to find the sweetness of who we are.

Tune into how you feel at the end of sessions. If you feel drained, then you probably were not tuned as optimally as you could have been, even though the session was not about you. You could reflect on how much safety, emotion, and wisdom you brought to the session so that you get the balance just right. It is, of course, a practice. It is not about getting it right each session. The practicing is the doing, session after session. Just as a pianist practices by playing, you are practicing how to be attuned properly and how you conduct yourself when you are doing the work.

20

PERMISSION TO BE WEIRD: THE CURE FOR THE WEARY THERAPIST

In this chapter, we discuss how to separate from clients after sessions and how not to get caught in a pattern of constantly responding to their demands. The cure is to be to find permission to be weird or to do things that are different in session. This sort of permission leads us directly to the heart of creativity.

Separating out from clients

I have long noticed a need for separating out from my clients and all their stuff. In session, I am with them and feel deeply into what they are going through. Yet, at the end of the session, or the end of the day, I need to let go of everything that I was holding for them. A long vacation is not going to cut it. I have needed ways of getting everybody, and all their demands, off of me and out of me. I have had to learn how to get clearer and more centered within myself so that I can really be present with clients day after day.

DOI: 10.4324/9781003283164-21

Just like any relationship, in therapy, there is a connection between therapist and client. We overlap with one another in a Venn diagram, where "you" and "me" merge into "we." As therapists, we can easily get caught up in our clients. We are interested in what is happening in their lives, and it can be easy to lose ourselves in them. We are impacted by our clients in healthy ways, yet we might also be affected in ways that drain us or make us stressed. Because of this danger of merging with our clients, it is important that we know how to separate ourselves out from them and have a clear enough delineation between our lives and theirs.

One easy way to create delineation is to get centered within ourselves. You might draw your attention within yourself. Where your point of awareness and attention lies is essentially where you live. Your life is where your attention is. In session, where is your attention? Is it entirely on your client? Is it somewhere lost in the content of the conversation? Or is some of your attention on you? Wherever you put your attention and awareness, that is where you reside.

Your awareness and attention might be in session with your client, yet it may also be on e-mails, what is going on at home, or on painful memories from the past. Maybe your attention is projected out into the future? Wherever it is, when you are with your client, you are paid for your attention. Part of your job is to be present in the moment with them, with your attention on the client and their presenting problem. We need to do this in a balanced way in order to have a sustainable practice.

When you are with your client, try practicing with one eye out and one eye in. Have part of your attention on the client and part of it within yourself. Your client does not need all of your attention and awareness entirely on them. It might feel too invasive and smothering for them. They also do not want your attention to be entirely out of the room either. They can feel it if you have something else going on. The goal is to find a way to have your attention and awareness centered on you so that your client can feel you and your presence without you invading their psychic space.

Nature abhors a vacuum. If you are in the client's space, then they are in your space. You would get all mixed in with the other one another, and that would become an enmeshed mess. When this happens, it is hard to know what is even happening or if therapy is even helping. The client may feel good because they are merging with you, but the best thing to do for them might be to have a clear delineation. There can be an agreement that says, "You are over there and I am over here, and I am not going to go into your space and you are not going to go into mine. Yet we are going to be together."

A new experience of connectedness

You are not abandoning the client if you do not look them directly in the eye the entire time. That is too intense. Instead, your point of awareness and attention can land softly right out in front of the client's face. They will feel like you are looking at them without it being too invasive of a gaze. The same goes for remote therapy, with your gaze softly out in front of you, not overly intent on the screen. If you imagine your attention gently landing right in front of the client's face or screen rather than peering straight into their eyes or the camera. It makes it easier to have your eyes gently focused in front of the client because you are present and aware but also not dialed into the client excessively.

If your client is having strong emotions and you start feeling those yourself, it may not serve them. The client might feel they have to start taking care of you or that their emotions are contagious. Conversely, if you were completely nonfeeling in the face of their strong emotions, then the client might not feel your empathy. A more neutral stance might instead be one in which you are a witness to their emotions and give your own reactions while not being overly responsible for their emotional state. In fact, if you are not overly responsible for their finding joy in life, it frees you up to be a more supportive presence. Perhaps you are partially responsible for the client being healthy and well, but ultimately it is their life, and you are just a caring, helpful part of it.

Neutrality is key to being an effective clinician. You can be on the same wavelength as the client, but you do not have to match them exactly where they are. You can be uniquely you, and they can be themselves, and you can still merge with one another. Nor do you need to match the client's affect, ideology, or the way they think about the world. You can meet them on the plane of human existence and then come back to your own personal life during and after session.

This sort of neutral stance may actually be optimal for the client's healing. Yet most people experience a sense of connectedness by merging and matching one another. It might not always be healthy, but most people feel connected when they mix in with one another emotionally and psychically. However, in therapy, we try to give them new experiences of connection that can feel deeply connected but not enmeshed and reactive. We try to show the client that we can empathize but not lose ourselves. We show them that we are with them but also give them some space. They are not alone, and we are not abandoning them.

This new way of relating might feel unfamiliar to the client, and you might have to explain a bit why you are being neutral. Perhaps you could say something like, "You may not have experienced me as warm and fuzzy at times, but I am still providing support, encouragement, and care. I don't say, 'oh, you poor thing' because I don't think that will help you. I do have a lot of compassion and empathy for what you are going through. I hope you experience me as empowering you."

Examining our programming

The notion that we might have more of our attention on ourselves in session rather than completely focused on the client might go against some of our training. We might have been trained to vacate ourselves in favor of being of service to the client. On a certain level, this training could be seen as a sort of program that controls us. It might dictate where we put our attention and awareness. The program might say that in order to be caring, we need to forget ourselves and sacrifice. It might say that being centered is self-centered.

On a sociological level, we can call this phenomenon conditioning or socializing. It runs us and dictates where we put our attention and awareness. Much like on a computer where there is a program that runs a set of operations, so too within ourselves, there might be programs that run our functioning. For instance, even though you might find it more compassionate and caring to tell a client that you care about them, a program from your training might say that it is counter-therapeutic to be that effusive. There can be all sorts of messages from your training that tell you what is caring or how to orient yourself in the world. It can be tremendously helpful to recognize how we are being controlled so we might be more creative and spontaneous in session.

Permission to change the coding

In computer programming, the way to get the system to change its operation is to change the input/output. The programmer needs to update the codes that tell the system what to do. Similarly, you could give yourself permission to change the coding and conditioning in the way that you practice. Might it be possible to generate your own sense of permission to not have to respond to every demand in session? Could you be more neutral in the face of the pulls and pushes in and around the therapy room?

If you have permission not to respond to everything, then others might experience you differently. It might throw them off a bit. They might experience it as weird. They might think you are weird. Your client might expect you to act in a predictable way. Yet when you don't, when your response is novel to them, it creates something new. It opens up a new pathway of relating that might be good. It might be healthy for them to be with somebody who is different and who is also, in a way, weird. Could you, as a therapist, have permission to be weird?

Resisting the pull to be normal

As a therapist, you have gotten along well because you have been able to fit in with life. You may have been effective because you have been, for the most part, agreeable and pleasant. It works to not be weird. It helps people feel safe with us. Weird is usually dangerous. Yet what if you could be safe but also have permission to be weird? What if you had permission not to run the expected social coding and instead could do something that is different or novel? Maybe you would find a genuine and authentic weirdness that comes from you. Maybe you would have permission to think differently, to express differently, to not get pulled into your clients' pain, and permission not to think about your clients after they leave the office.

When you give yourself permission to do something different, you open up the possibility for creativity. When we do something creative, it stays with the client. We need permission first in order to be creative – the permission to do something different needs to come first. Then we might say something unexpected that could stay with the client for days or even years to come. This is the heart of creativity in our work.

There is such a pull to have a normative experience with clients where the interaction is socially appropriate, yet that is not necessarily healing. We have to resist that pull. We have to actively find our own voice and not be what we think a therapist is *supposed* to be. Instead of saying something predictably soothing, maybe we could find a gentle way to challenge the client. It would be interesting to see what happens for us if we have permission to be centered, to not respond to everybody's demands, and to be creative with the client. If therapy can be a place where we can create new possibilities, then the client can then do things that are creative and different in their life as well.

Bonus exercise: Awareness meditation

In order to get comfortable with a more centered and grounded way of working in session, it can help to practice being centered and grounded in your daily life. An awareness meditation can be a way of practicing being centered and grounded. Meditation has been a vehicle for personal growth and development for ages, and it does not need to be religious or spiritual in order to practice. Below is an awareness meditation that you might use in your daily life to help you be more centered in your sessions.

Directions:

Get comfortable in a chair. Take a moment to check in with yourself. Notice where your attention has been. Notice where your awareness has been. What are you getting caught up in psychologically and emotionally? Where has the demand on your attention been? Are there people or places your awareness is more focused on these days?

Visualization:

Imagine your attention like points scattered all over time and space. These points of attention are in people, in projects, and in clients. They are in the past and in the future. You are up to a pretty big life so you likely have points of awareness and attention all over the place, which is great. Just for a moment, see what you experience when you to pull all of your attention and awareness out of all things external and call your attention and awareness back to you.

Notice:

What does it feel like to have your awareness, your attention, in you, on you, inside of you? There is nothing else to attend to right now, your awareness and your attention is centered on you. It is okay if your mind goes all over the place, but your awareness is inside of you, in this moment. If you are noticing any tension, stress, or other people's attention inside of you, ask that that be moved out, just for a moment.

Clearing:

Get everybody's attention, their demand on you, out of you. Separate them out for a moment. You have called your attention and awareness out of everyone else and everything else, out of the past and the future, and brought it back to here and now. As you take up residence within yourself, if there are other things within you, other people's awareness in you (clients, family members, loved ones, demands from business, work, relationships), let that fall away from you for a little bit. For this moment, you do not have to manage or handle anybody else's demands. Just stay centered on you.

Breathing:

Take a few breaths and see how this feels. Stay here as long as you would like. When you are ready, you can come out of this visualization into normal waking consciousness but remain centered within yourself.

The idea in this meditation is that you can find yourself caught up in all sorts of other things such as people, activities, and clients. You can be in the past and the future, as your attention and awareness might be caught up there. Just as you are elsewhere in other things, other things are in you. This is pretty normal for all of us to be mixed in like this. Yet being a clinician and getting deeply mixed into many other people's lives, it becomes hazardous. We need to cleanse out or clear out everyone else at the end of the session or at the end of the day.

21

ACCESSING YOUR HIGHER WISDOM

This chapter addresses what it means to access your higher wisdom. This is the part of ourselves that has information and gets a deep sense of instant knowing. Some people report experiencing their higher wisdom as a download, others as insights coming from some channel within themselves. Others say that it shows up by communicating through pictures and metaphors. Whatever the form of your higher wisdom, learning how to access and use it is the key to accelerated development as a clinician.

Accessing your higher wisdom

One key question for new and old therapists alike is to ask ourselves, "How much do I actually know?" How much do our training and life experience inform us when it comes to helping clients? There is an aspect of our work for which it is beneficial to come from a place of not knowing because it honors the mysteries of life. Life is mysterious,

DOI: 10.4324/9781003283164-22

people are mysterious, and we should not set ourselves up as having all of the answers to all of life's questions.

If we come from a place of complete unknowing, however, as if we have no information, then we do our clients a disservice, and we withhold some of the gifts we have to give. If a client asks for advice about a certain situation in their life, then we might help guide them. We want to give the client a little bit of information or wisdom so that they can find their way. To do so, you do not necessarily need to develop more knowledge or get more training (although that wouldn't hurt). You just need to grow more confidence in what you already know within you.

It helps to define and clarify where your inherent knowing comes from. One sort of knowing comes from having studied a topic or learned from a mentor. This is essential in our field and gives us a solid footing with our clinical approach. Another sort of knowing comes from lived experience. This knowing might be a felt sense of something resonating as true or an intuitive understanding inside yourself. You have had experiences in your life that shape what you know.

The knowing you have from experience can certainly be brought into your sessions right away. For example, if you have a child and a client asks you a parenting question, you might have some information and answers based on your experience. It could just be your answer for your situation and not something that is applicable to everyone. You may be able to relate and give the clients a sense of what has worked for you. But what are you supposed to do about situations where you do not have knowing from studying a topic or from lived experience? Your training and reading, nor your lived experience may not have told you what to do or say in session. In those cases, you need to tap into something more intuitive within yourself.

This is a leap into something more abstract and right-brained, but if you are able to access an intuitive knowing, or higher wisdom, inside yourself, then it can be your quickest way to develop as a clinician. Otherwise, it is going to take a lifetime of studying and lived experience for you to get to a place of confidence with what you know. To be effective sooner rather than later, you have to find some way to feel comfortable with what you know within you and be able to bring that into the room. In the very beginning of your training, when you knew very little about counseling, you had to rely on this sort of knowing. You had the wisdom of knowing what to say that would soothe and comfort the client even if you didn't have the answers to their problems.

I am training a new therapist whose client came in recently and disclosed for the first time a traumatic event from her childhood. The therapist, upon hearing the client's disclosure, could not say, "Hold on a moment while I get my book about trauma." In the moment, the therapist had to access some wisdom about what to say and do in the session. They had never experienced a client disclosing trauma before, and while the therapist knew some basic information about trauma-informed care, they had to tap into an innate sense of how to work with another human being disclosing something painful from their past.

The information that the therapist had within themselves in that moment is something that is there from the very beginning. It does not go away. It stays with us, and if you learn how to tap into your higher wisdom, you may find it to be your biggest gift as a clinician.

What higher wisdom looks like

Higher wisdom does not come from book learning or classroom experience. It emanates from the creative part of the mind that is open to free association. You might find this part of your mind saying to your client in session, "I have no idea where this is coming from," but then you take a risk and share an intuitive insight that resonates with the client.

Your insight can show up like a flash of inspiration in your mind. Or it will be like downloading a file of information. Whatever the feeling, it is much different from the information you receive from the analytical part of your mind. That part can get in the way, and try to make sense of everything that is being spoken in session. If we can ask the analyst to step aside a bit and leave room for downloads of insight and flashes of inspiration to occur, then we can find new possibilities in therapy. These shimmers of insight are there every session if you are willing to be open to them. They show up as right-brained, mental image pictures.

Your analyzing, rational mind can work in balance with the higher wisdom aspect. The analyst can do the work of gathering information, considering interventions, and making hypotheses, while the right-brained, higher wisdom part of your mind tunes into your client like a radio dial. Your wisdom can communicate with your rational mind through mental images that emerge within the conversation in session. You can take those mental images, pull some information out of them, and interpret them like a dream, communicating them to your client. Perhaps you have an idea or image that pops into your mind through your higher wisdom. You could simply just share that image or idea with the client. Yet it becomes even more effective when you are able to take the information you gather from the mental image picture and work it into the flow of the conversation.

Bringing one's higher information gracefully into the session is an art. It is a balancing act, with one eye trained inward on yourself and one eye looking out at the client. In order to safely tap into your own innate higher wisdom, you can follow these two steps.

Step one: Creating safety in your body

If you want to have access to more information in session, then you need to get safe in your body. Intuitive information shows up in the body. If you are not there to receive it, then it becomes challenging to bring it into your sessions. If your attention is not in your body, then you might not be at home to receive the insight and inspiration coming from your wise mind. Instead, you become an ungrounded, disembodied talking head. You could still do great work this way, yet it is likely much harder, and the work goes more slowly. Instead, being safely grounded and centered in your body, you can get access to higher wisdom which moves much more quickly.

You just have to trust and allow yourself not to have that next thing figured out in session or be planning the next intervention you want to say. You have to trust that when it's time for you to say something, that you will find what is needed. The key is to have your attention within your body and be listening in a way that allows for creative insight and inspiration to emerge. You may not need to listen as hard to every word and every sentence that the client says. Doing so may leave you too intently focused on the content of the session. Instead, listening more skillfully to the music of the session, not the words, helps.

The music is within each client, but you have to tune into it. You need to take some space while the client is talking and sit back a little bit and listen more deeply. Get more clear within yourself where you want to go, and then figure out how to weave your insights into the conversation. The client wants us to tune into what is really going on with them. To do this, we need to stay in touch with our own body, listen deeply, and respond from a place of trust in our own wisdom.

Step two: Trusting your higher wisdom

If the therapist trusts whatever comes up in their mind and follows what it compels them to say or do, then the client will feel held and guided in ways that are different from being with a therapist who is just operating from their intellectual knowing. The therapy moves more quickly and more efficiently when higher wisdom is involved. Trusting your wisdom is the next step after getting safe in your body. We can start by understanding where we might have stopped learning to trust our own wisdom in the first place and started doubting what we know.

Most of us trusted our intuition when we were little kids. Back then, we freely shared what we were thinking and feeling without doubting it. Yet over time, we were socialized to question what we innately know. We were taught instead to look outside of ourselves for information. Our own knowing is often judged or invalidated. It was likely questioned by teachers, colleagues, classmates, or parents.

For example, a young child might say to a bully at school, "I don't like you," because something does not feel right to them in the interaction with the other child. They may be quickly admonished because it is not nice and it might hurt the bully's feelings. Now the child is confused. Something did not feel right to the child about the bully, but others are telling them that it is not okay to say so. We have all been conditioned in some way not to believe or speak our own knowing.

Our knowing has been whacked and invalidated in this way. There is some healing to be done in your relationship with your own higher wisdom. If all of the layers of conditioning you have been carrying were stripped away, then you would be left with your natural state of mind, which is beautiful and glowing. Clients want to be around that kind of radiance. But, like most of us, you may have accumulated all sorts of conditioning along the way. If you walk into session like Pigpen from *Peanuts*, full of dust and thoughts and feelings and reactions, your sessions will not go so smoothly. You will get in your own way by overthinking and trying to make sense of everything your client says. Instead, if you get grounded in your body and trust your intuition again, then your sessions will shine.

CONCLUSION

Being a therapist is the perfect artform. It is a living expression of who we are and takes a lifetime to master. Being a therapist provides continual opportunities for growth and development. Just when you think that you might have a solid sense of what to do clinically, the practice of therapy can change on you and throw a curveball.

You have to adapt and be ready for anything when you are a therapist. The context in which we practice is constantly changing, and we need to guard against becoming set in our ways. We will continually be learning about human nature and how to best help one another evolve. Like climbing a mountain without a top, we must be prepared to constantly reach for new heights, as the potential for growth never stops.

I remember when I became aware that I had found my life's calling as a therapist. I was sitting in session in a plain clinic room at The Family Institute at Northwestern University. It was an individual session with an adult client, and we were making some sort of breakthrough. I can't remember the content of the conversation, as it was back when I was in my second year of graduate school. Yet I do recall the feeling in that room. The client was making a connection to some answer or resolution of a problem that had been bothering them. I recall the sense of relief

DOI: 10.4324/9781003283164-23

and euphoria that the client was feeling as he talked his way into an understanding about his life.

In that moment, I felt myself drifting a bit. I was really committed to the session, overly eager perhaps as a therapist in training, yet something pulled me up and outside of my body. I floated out of the room, above the building, and into the parking lot outside. I recall gazing over the head of the client into that parking lot at dusk and connecting to a deep sense that I had found my life's purpose. I knew then that I wanted to be there for these moments in people's lives when they found insight into themselves. I wanted to be a part of those *aha* moments and feel the euphoria and relief as life's dramas are beautifully resolved. I wanted to help create opportunities for people to find their truth.

It was so clear to me in that clinic room in 2005. I knew that I was going to be a therapist for the rest of my life. It was euphoric and relieving for me as well to find what I was meant to do. I was aware as it was happening that it was a privilege to find my life's work. Many people do not have that freedom to discover what they love and are meant to do. For me, it was the resolution of so much hard work within myself, resolving my own wounds. I felt myself stepping into being a "wounded healer." As I healed my own emotional, psychological, and relational wounds, I cooked up a sort of medicine within myself. I was becoming a medicine carrier of sorts, bringing compassion and care to the other wounded human beings around me.

Coming into my body from floating out in that parking lot and back into the clinic room, I connected again to what the client was talking about and I probably offered some sort of support and encouragement for them to keep going. I had a pen and paper at my side table at the time, and I wrote down a note to myself. The note really wasn't clinical in nature, but it was certainly inspired by the content of that session. It read, "Who I am informs my work. My work informs who I am."

I try to take that note into sessions every day. It is precisely who I am that informs, uplifts, and carries the clinical work. The clinical work also informs, reveals, and elicits who I am. If I am paying attention, I learn a little something about myself each session. The clients teach us about ourselves as they share who they are with us. It is a sacred undertaking and a humbling gift to have found therapy. I hope that you feel the same way.

When times are stressful, it can be challenging to connect to the heart of what it means to be a therapist in this way. My moment of floating in reverie while discovering my life's work can feel so far away today amidst the daily stress of seeing client after client. Oftentimes, it feels much more like a job than a sacred gift. Feeling ineffective, letting clients down, missing the mark with interpretations, and watching our clients continually struggle is part of the work, even for the most experienced clinicians.

Connecting back to the roots of why we do what we do can help us get through the tough times. Can you recall or connect back to when you knew that you wanted to be a therapist? Can you remember some of those first clients that solidified for you that this is what you are meant to do? I remember my first clients, and in addition to my soaring moments early in my training, I recall vivid early struggles and how they shaped me. Connecting to our early growing pains can be just as revitalizing as remembering our first successes.

I clearly remember how it felt to run my first therapy group. It was a men's group that I had put together in the final semester of graduate school. Composed of a few of my male clients along with some colleagues' clients, this men's group was my first experience of taking in all the stimuli and data from a therapy process group. I was tracking what one man was saying while noticing another who was checked out and another who wanted to interrupt. I could sense the undercurrent anxieties in the room and overlapping stories that the men were bringing to the group. It was way too much for me to handle and I became overwhelmed, not knowing what to address. There was silence in the room, and the six group members looked to me to say something. A small bead of sweat dripped down the inside of my arm, and I panicked.

That men's group was not the first time I felt that level of panic and overwhelm as a new clinician, but it was one of the most formative. With the pressure of an entire group waiting for me to lead them, I had to find something to say. I had to pull on something from within myself. I had to synthesize all the information in the group and consult to some aspect of it.

I don't remember what I said in that moment, but I recall how I had to summon grace under pressure and find trust in myself. I had to jump into the unknown and say something. It is that sort of leap into the unknown that waits for us today in each therapy session. We may not burst into a sweat, but there are plenty of times of not knowing what to do and then summoning some insight or intervention to try to take the process forward.

Looking back to early, formative experiences, I know that my supervisors at the time were strongly holding me up while I learned. It was their belief in me and their guidance that helped me have the confidence to try new things and find my voice as a clinician. It is the supervisor who plays such a key role in uncovering the therapist that lies within the student. They not only teach us how to do the work and manage cases, they also nurture our abilities and nourish our souls when we feel lost or exhausted.

It is no mistake that here at the conclusion of this book that, we are focusing on formative clinical moments and early supervisors. Those nascent experiences shape us and might be the key to future growth. They help us start out on the track of becoming a therapist and are the pathways back when we get lost. When we get stuck today, we can look back on what helped us early on and remember those lessons so that we can reinvent our practices again. Reconnecting to real supervision at a soul level, we can believe in ourselves again.

This is the message to take going forward. When you are stuck, lost, overwhelmed, or burnt out, look back to why you became a therapist in the first place. Find the supervisor, professor, or mentor who got through to you. Connect with them in your heart, and reconnect to the soul of this work.

I also invite you to take a blessing going forward. I wish for you a real sense of purpose in your work. I invite you to regularly recognize the difference that you make in the lives of your clients. Your compassion and healing spread forth to their lives and into the lives of those around them. Your loving kindness blesses your clients and the world they live in. It flows into the subtext of society and makes our world a gentler and saner place to live.

I invite you to find real joy in your work. Instead of being caught up in our heads, overthinking therapy, we should make ourselves the musical instrument of change. We bring forth the music of therapy in session by becoming more of who we are day by day. I wish for you to discover that it is simply by being who you are, here in this world, that you make all the difference. May your clinical practice be an expression of who you are ... a work of art. May your sessions flow like music into the hearts of others, and may you find joy, meaning, and purpose in the soul of therapy.

INDEX